WALKING
in the
MIRACULOUS

MY HEALING JOURNEY THROUGH CANCER

AMANDA HUNT

Published by Silversmith Press, Houston, Texas.

Silversmith Press titles may be purchased in bulk for educational, business, fundraising, or sales promotional use. For information, please email office@silversmithpress.com.

Any internet addresses, phone numbers, company or product information printed in this book are offered as a resource and are not intended in any way to be or to imply an endorsement by the author and/or publisher, nor does the author/publisher vouch for the existence, content or services of these sites, phone numbers, companies or products beyond the life of this book.

ISBN 978-1-7378859-6-2 (Softcover Book)
ISBN 978-1-7378859-7-9 (eBook)

Silversmith Press, Houston, Texas–www.silversmithpress.com
Printed in the United States of America.

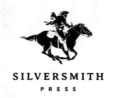

SILVERSMITH
PRESS

This book is dedicated to my children:
Cameron, Courtney, Chelsea, Alaina and Jacob.
You all bring immeasurable joy to my life.

Children are a gift from the Lord. A reward from Him.
Psalm 127:3

Contents

Acknowledgments

First of all, I want to thank the Lord for healing me. Thank You, God, for being true to Your Word and for fulfilling Your promises. Thank You for never leaving me or forsaking me. Thank You for the gift of life, the gift of healing, and for giving me a future with my family. Your mercies amaze me over and over again. I'm thankful You can read my heart because my words could never come close to thanking You enough for what You've done for me and my family.

I would also like to thank the many people who have had a role in my healing journey.

To my husband, Jonathan-Thank you for joining me in this spiritual warfare, for leading us in prayer and communion, and constantly encouraging me. You never once showed fear and never once spoke doubt. I couldn't have made it through this journey without you. Thank you for being a strong, supportive husband, spiritual leader and my safe place. I can always count on you. You are exactly who I prayed for when I prayed for a husband and you are a gift straight from God.

I will always love and adore you with every beat of my heart.

Cameron—You are so full of joy and laughter, it's contagious. I can always count on you to make me laugh and smile. I love your humor and your sweet personality. God has gifted you with a unique joy and sweetness that blesses me. I love you so much! Thank you for bringing a special joy to every day.

Courtney—You are a peacemaker and always love others above yourself. What a gift you are, especially in such a large family. Thank you for your willingness to help when I needed you the most. You are a natural leader, mature beyond your years, and an inspiration to me. You have a beautiful heart that blesses everyone around you. I love you!

Chelsea—You are so full of love and I appreciate that you always give so much affection. Your hugs and snuggles were exactly what I needed on many of those hard days. I love you tons and I love your comforting hugs every day. I also love that you are all things fancy and I can always count on you to be my shopping partner. Thank you for the abundance of love that shines through you.

Alaina—You are such a sweet joy. Your sweet personality and your humor always bring a smile to my face. You light up every room you enter and I'm thankful for the happiness you bring to our entire family. I love that you always have a worship song on your heart and your songs always encourage me. I love you, baby girl.

Jacob—My sweet baby boy, you have brought so much joy and purpose into my life. Your fun loving personality just melts my heart. God knew that I needed the love of a baby during this season. I love you and I'm so thankful for you.

Grandma Hunt—You are a treasure. Thank you for fighting for my life. You taught me a new way of praying and taking authority over my health. Thank you for your willingness to share, pray, and speak the promises of God. You took me under your wing and you have become one of my closest friends. I love you.

Nickie—You were involved in every step of this journey. Thank you for speaking life over me, anointing me, praying for me daily, and allowing the Holy Spirit to speak through you. You are bold, you are a fierce prayer warrior, and you fought for my life. I can never thank you enough. Your friendship is a gift from God.

Dolly–Thank you for praying fervently and standing in agreement with me. You are a dear friend and I appreciate all of the love and support from you and your family. You have been a true blessing.

Mr. Lee–Thank you for your willingness to share your testimony. Your support and encouragement were especially helpful because you were the only person I knew who truly understood my situation. Thank you for your guidance and for believing I would see a miracle. You have inspired me to follow in your steps by openly sharing my testimony as well.

Pastor Lonnie–I am thankful for the atmosphere that you have cultivated in Christ Central Church, where the Spirit of God is welcome to move and miracles can take place. Many times, God would speak directly to my situation through your sermons, so thank you for always being obedient to speak the Word of God. Not only did you personally take the time to check on us and pray for us, but you have equipped a community of leaders within our home church so that I had a support system I could turn to for prayer as well. I am so thankful to have such an amazing pastor and attend the most incredible church ever!

Manning–You are an incredibly talented, generous,

and sweet hair stylist. Thank you for making me feel beautiful for pictures. I am very blessed to be one of your clients.

Aleck–Photo shoots with you are so much fun! Thank you for your time, creativity, and flexibility to take pictures for this book. You are incredibly talented. I am very fortunate to have found such an amazing photographer. You will go far in life.

Joanna–You are the most amazing and patient publisher. Thank you for helping me turn my manuscript into a book and for honoring my vision. You were so patient and encouraging to me in every step of the process. It has truly been a pleasure working with you.

Chris–Thank you for taking my vision and bringing the book cover to life. It is absolutely perfect! Well done!

Nicole–Thank you for carrying the joy of the Lord in the oncology office. You are a light. Thank you for giving me the opportunity to share my testimony in the prayer group; I'm so grateful for you.

Jackie–You spoke a prophetic word over my life, including "You will write the book." Thank you for following the prompting of the Holy Spirit. This book would not exist without that confirmation.

To all of our friends and family who prayed, encouraged us and helped us out with the kids, we appreciate every one of you. Thank you for your love and support during the most challenging time of our lives.

Sincerely,
Amanda

Introduction

Are you or someone you love experiencing hope-lessness because of a medical diagnosis? Maybe it's recent, and you don't even know where to begin, or perhaps you've been battling something for a while, and you find yourself feeling weary. Let me tell you; you are not alone. I've been there. I've felt the blow of the words from a doctor that shake you to your core. I've felt the fear, the loneliness, the struggle, the un-certainty. But I've also felt what it's like to be on the other side of a fatal diagnosis. I've felt the joy and freedom of walking in the miraculous, of seeing the Word of God come to pass in my life.

If you had asked me on the day of my diagnosis if I could ever be thankful for this journey, there's not a chance I would have said yes; I would have done any-thing to avoid it. Because of what I have experienced, now I am overjoyed that I have faced the unimag-inable and have a testimony of God's faithfulness. Now, I want to share my experience to help you on your journey. You aren't walking alone, and while I can't be with you physically, I am with you in spirit. I am praying for you because I am praying for every person who picks up this book. I may not know your name, but rest assured, God does. He holds your pain; He bottles your tears and counts them as precious. He loves you, and He wants to show Himself strong on your behalf. There is no distance in the spirit. Even though I am not with you, God is, and my prayer is that as you read this book, you will know His love in a new way and sense Him closer than the air you breathe.

When I began my healing journey, I was overwhelmed and didn't know where to start. I do well with organized to-do lists, concrete plans, and order. I am a mother of five, with triplets in the mix, so if our lives and schedules aren't in order, chaos will surely ensue. As you might imagine, when I got my diagnosis, everything concrete in my life seemed to vanish in thin air. I didn't know where to turn, even though I was, and am a woman of faith. I'd had difficulty in my life, but nothing like this. There wasn't exactly a guidebook or a tutorial on "How to Get Healed by God," and this isn't one either. Healing is very much an individual spiritual journey of faith and obedience to His leading. The healing journey is not going to look the same for everyone since we are all unique individuals with different needs on different journeys. But through this book, I want to take you along my journey of receiving a miraculous healing and the lessons I learned along the way. I want to help you find encouragement, hope, and inspiration no matter what you may be facing. In this book, I am going to share what God says in His Word and challenge you to speak His promises. My faith was stretched and tested as I believed God for what He promised, and yours will be too. I will also offer suggestions and assignments to help you keep your focus on the promises of God, so you can overcome the lies of the enemy.

I know that my story, my testimony, is not just for me. God brought me through this so I can live as an example and encouragement to you and anyone who needs a miracle from God. I want to see you walking in the miraculous, and God does too! I believe wholeheartedly that God wants to show up in your circumstances. I believe that as we all take hold of the truth of His Word, we will see healing testimonies multiplied exponentially! Yes, God spared me and healed me so His glory can be revealed. This I know: If He did it for me, He can do it for you. As you read this book, hold that truth close to your heart and join me in walking in the miraculous.

CHAPTER ONE

The Diagnosis

August of 2021 started out as a pretty amazing month. The world was opening up and my husband and I decided to book a vacation to my favorite place on earth, Oahu, Hawaii. As a Florida native, I love the sunshine, but anyone who knows me well would agree that I was born on the wrong side of the earth. Half of my heart belongs to beautiful Hawaii! The trip was scheduled for December of the same year, which seemed like an eternity away at the time. Travel rates were reasonable, and that would give me more time to prepare myself to leave our youngest son, who was just one at the time, for an extended period. We have a family of seven and a jam-packed schedule, so my husband, Jonathan, and I were very excited for quality time together, just the two of us. We were still newlyweds essentially, married in 2018 when Jonathan became a full-time dad to my four little girls. Getting alone time together is important for us to keep our marriage first. Little did I know what we were about to endure prior to this vacation. I would soon realize that God had a hand in every detail of our lives, including the planning of this trip!

August is my birthday month, so I always schedule my annual health exam then. I had missed my post-partum checkup after the birth of our son, so I was long overdue for an exam. I went to my appointment expecting just another routine visit I could check off my list. That day, I was feeling a little impatient because Jonathan was home watching all five kids so I could have some time to myself. I could not wait to go shopping at the mall after my appointment. These annual exams are never pleasant but generally pretty quick. It seemed to take longer than usual, and I was doing my best to endure it. Just then, my doctor said in a very flat tone, "There is a growth on your cervix. I need to do a biopsy to see what it is." I couldn't believe what I just heard. My heart sank, and fearful thoughts immediately flooded my mind as I struggled to hold back the tears. The doctor didn't really say anything after that. He just proceeded with the biopsy and assured me he would call as soon as the results were back.

I was still in disbelief when I went home and told

Jonathan what had happened. He did his best to calm my nerves and reminded us both that there was no need to worry until we knew for sure what it was. As the days passed, part of me was enjoying blissful ignorance, and the other part was dreading confirmation that something was wrong. Every time the phone rang, my heart would pound out of my chest. Then finally, a week later, on Thursday, August 26th, 2021, I was standing in my kitchen when the phone rang, and the caller ID showed it was my doctor's office. I can still remember my heart pounding so hard I thought it might jump out of my chest, my hands absolutely drenched in sweat as my emotions and nerves took control. As I answered, I immediately ran past my children, firmly instructing them to stay inside the house. I went outside to where Jonathan was doing yard work, then put the doctor on speakerphone. He informed me he had the results back. Jonathan and I just looked at each other as the words came out of the speaker.

"You have cancer," he said.

Before my mind could even process it, my body reacted. I was physically trembling in fear, crying, and completely freaking out. I felt crushed, terrified, confused, shocked, and sad. I don't know if I could put words to every emotion I experienced in that moment and in the months to follow. I believed that my doctor was telling me the truth, although I was in a state of complete disbelief. I told the doctor that I needed to see it; I needed the results uploaded to my online patient portal right away. I hoped to find a mistake. I thought, *maybe he is looking at the wrong patient chart, or reading it wrong. How could this happen to me?* My mind was racing.

I struggled to hear his words, "I am going to refer you to an oncologist. I will give her a call myself to make sure you get scheduled in quickly. We will need to start with a radical hysterectomy."

I heard his words, but could barely comprehend them. I felt a heaviness, and like my throat was closing. I could hardly breathe, much less speak. He told me that the cancer was found in the outer cervix, but that is not where they believed it originated. He spoke the usual doctor dialogue, "We won't know anything more until you have additional testing done. I am also going to refer you for a CT."

With every word he spoke, my heart and mind seemed to leave my control. I wondered if I could have a heart attack at that moment. As he continued in "doctor speak," I leaned over the fence behind me, grasping for something concrete as I tried to control my thoughts. I had overcome major trauma in my life before, but nothing like this. I equated a cancer diagnosis with a death sentence. I immediately thought of my family. I was not ready to die and leave my children behind. They need me, and my husband needs me too. I thought of the outcome of that surgery, *what if they could not get all the cancer out? What if it had spread? How far could it spread? Where did it originate? Why is this in my body?* My mind was flooded with fears and "what-ifs." I cried so many tears. Waves of grief and fear hit me over and over. Little did I know that this was just the beginning of the battle in my mind.

The phone call must have lasted under five minutes, but the dialogue of thoughts blasting in my mind made it seem like an eternity. After the call, I collapsed into my husband's arms sobbing. We both agreed that the children should not know anything about this at this point. We could barely comprehend it ourselves; how could we break this kind of news to our precious, innocent little children? It was a burden they did not need to bare. I was not able to handle my own grief and fears, so how could I comfort them? No, we weren't going to burden them with the fear and uncertainty until we had more answers. We allowed ourselves a few more minutes outside, but the kids needed dinner, baths, and help with homework. I had to "suck it up" as they say, put on a happy face, and get on with being a mom for the evening so that my children would be okay. But, I knew that emotionally I was not okay. I needed someone to talk to for support. As I made dinner that evening, I remembered a testimony I heard about an elder in our church named Mr. Lee. He had been diagnosed with a very rare cancer that almost took his life. The doctors gave him only weeks to live, and the cancer was so rare and aggressive that he couldn't even find an oncologist who was able to see him within the expected lifespan he was given. However, the Holy Spirit spoke to him and confirmed that he would be healed. He was miraculously healed, and to this day, he shares his testimony, glorifying God and encouraging others. As I thought about it, I knew I must speak with him.

The next day, my results were uploaded to my online patient portal, and it made me sick to look at them. The biopsy indicated poorly differentiated (high grade) adenocarcinoma of the cervix, favoring endocervical origin, which is not quite where it was found. I immediately began questioning God. *How could this be His plan for me?* It didn't make any sense, not after all He had done to get me to where I am today. *Was this a punishment? I have done some terrible things in my life, and the wages of sin is death, so did I do something to deserve this?* Even though the questions rolled through my mind, in my heart I didn't really believe that cancer was from God. It couldn't be. I thought of the many biblical promises I've heard over and over throughout my life. Jeremiah 29 tells us that His plans are good, so why is this happening? My thoughts were like a roller coaster. I did not want the radical surgery, but I also didn't want to neglect my health and die. When I turned 38 exactly one week prior, it seemed so old, but suddenly, 38 was incredibly young. In that moment, looking at those biopsy results, something rose up in my spirit. I decided that I was not dying yet, and I was not going down without a fight. I was not accepting surgery as the only option without trusting in God first. My resolve was clear, but at the same time, I wondered, *was that too risky?* After all, this was cancer. But I didn't want to mutilate my body. I wanted my body to remain whole; I wanted to remain a whole woman. I wanted cancer to be gone. In all my uncertainty, one thing I knew for sure was that God "could" heal me. I didn't doubt His ability. He's the God who created the heavens and the earth, formed us from dust, parted the Red Sea, caused water to spring up from a rock, healed the leper, and made the blind to see and the lame to walk. I could go on and on about the miraculous things He has done! No matter how many times I read or hear about the miracles in the Bible, they never grow any less fascinating. I know what He can do. I know there's nothing that He can't do! The question I struggled with initially was, *will He do it for me?*

I did not know the answer, but I decided to put my faith in Him anyway because only He could do what I needed. Jonathan and I agreed—this would be another testimony to strengthen our faith and our children's faith. We chose to believe that God was going to heal me! Yes, it was a choice. We had two options: we could either accept the report of the doctor or the report of the Lord. In the natural, this seemed slightly crazy. After all, I only personally knew of one person healed of cancer years ago, and that was Mr. Lee. I didn't even know him personally; I had just heard his story talked about at church over the years. I am so grateful he openly shared his testimony because it became an anchor of hope for me. Because Mr. Lee was willing to share his testimony, I was encouraged by it. I wanted to be healed and encourage others with my testimony too. Sharing your testimony is so important because you never know who God will place in your path who needs to hear it and be encouraged by it.

Three days after my diagnosis, I was at church and saw Mr. Lee. I asked if we could talk after service, and he agreed. He was kind and compassionate, and full of faith. The wisdom he shared was crucial for my journey. The first piece of advice he gave me was "Be careful who you tell. Cancer is a written and spoken curse that you have to break." He taught me to say out loud, "I break the curse of cancer spoken over me. I break the curse of cancer written over me. I do not receive this diagnosis. Cancer is not mine." He also talked to me about the power of forgiveness, but I had so many things on my mind, I didn't fully grasp what he was communicating until later on in my journey. I took in as much as I could, and I was so grateful. Mr. Lee was one of the first people to believe with us and pray for the miracle that we sought. I'll always be thankful for his example and compassion. Throughout this journey, he was in touch with us and understood the battle I faced in my mind. He always encouraged Jonathan and me, continually pointing us toward what God said and not the doctors. I also especially appreciate how he reached out to support Jonathan individually and help him as he was supporting me. I still can't imagine how difficult this was for Jonathan.

That first meeting with Mr. Lee was two weeks before my CT appointment, but it felt like an eternity of waiting, and I spent a lot of time in prayer. We only shared our story with a few pastors and people who we knew were serious about prayer. We trusted these friends not to spread the news or speak negative words of doubt over us. The Bible says in James 5:14–15, "Is any among you sick? Let him call for the elders of the church, and let them pray over him, anointing him with oil in the Name of the Lord. And the prayer of faith will save the sick, and the Lord will raise him up. And if he has committed sins, he will be forgiven." We had a very small group of close friends who we knew would truly stand in faith with us, pray earnestly and not spread the news.

One morning, my husband's grandmother, Grandma Hunt, stopped by our house to drop off a birthday card for Jonathan. I had no plans to tell her what was happening because we did not want to have the news accidentally leaked to other family members. She wasn't planning to stay long so we stood at the door chatting for a moment and she began speaking an encouraging word about our future. I knew it was God-inspired. She had no idea that I was wrestling with dark thoughts, wondering if I even had a future. I decided that we needed to tell her because we needed her help and encouragement.

Grandma Hunt has served Jesus nearly her entire life and has experienced miracle after miracle. She is a fierce woman of prayer and she is known for being very sensitive to the Holy Spirit. When Grandma Hunt says, "The Lord spoke something to me," we all know to listen! She is a treasure to have in our family and we are grateful for her.

Grandma Hunt was about to turn to leave, and I asked her if she would come to the family room for a private chat with Jonathan and me, away from the children. As we sat down, I burst into tears and began to tell her about the call from my doctor and the diagnosis I had received. I barely got the words out of my mouth as she immediately blurted out, "That's a lie!" I was a little confused at first, but she continued, "That's a lie from the enemy. You do not have cancer. Jesus already paid the price for that; it is not yours. Let's pray right now." She began to pray with Jonathan and me. She spoke words of healing and proclaimed the biblical inheritance we have because of the sacrifice of Jesus. She cursed cancer and told it to leave and never come back. She encouraged us not to believe this diagnosis. She reminded us that Satan is a liar, a thief, and this is an attack from him, not God. She instructed us to start taking communion while seeking healing. Her visit was so encouraging, I continued to cry even after she left, so thankful that God had sent her our way. The decision to share my story with her would not only prove to be a wise one, but it also connected me to her in a new way as we became closer and closer over the following months.

That night after she left, we decided to take communion as she suggested. We did not have any unleavened bread, which is normally used, but we made do with what we had. Jonathan pulled out a small plate and placed two pinches of butter bread on it. Then he poured a few sips of red wine into a small glass. We sat down awkwardly in the living room, just staring at it. We had taken communion many times at church, with our pastor leading and beautiful worship music playing in the background, but never on our own. We did not know how to do it ourselves, but we were desperate and willing to put our pride aside to try anything. Grandma had shown us in scripture how the Lord commanded all of His children to "do this in remembrance of Him" (Luke 22:19). We looked at each other and giggled at our awkwardness and decided to at least put on some worship music. Then we said a prayer and partook of the communion elements. There was nothing spectacular that happened in that moment. It was an act of sheer obedience to Jesus' command in scripture. It was us surrendering our will and pride over to the Lord. I felt shy and embarrassed to take communion with Jonathan and make declarations in faith. I didn't want to pray and cry out loud in front of him or look weird. But I was desperate enough to try anything. Neither of us knew what to say, but we figured it out.

After a few nights of taking communion together, we became more and more comfortable with it, enjoying it as part of our nightly routine. It became a very sacred time of peace and comfort to our hearts that we prioritized and looked forward to. For us, our communion prayer would begin by thanking God for who He is and the relationship we have with Him. We would always thank Him for allowing His only Son to be beaten and bruised for our iniquities as we would take the bread. Then we would thank Him for shedding His blood as we would take a sip of the wine. We recalled God's own Word back to Him by declaring His healing promises. I would declare, "By Your stripes, I am healed. I curse cancer like Jesus cursed the fig tree, I command it to wither up and die. In the Name and authority of Jesus Christ, I command cancer to leave my body. My body is a temple of the Holy Spirit, and cancer cannot stay. The price has already been paid. Sickness does not belong to me, I give it back to Jesus, the one who already defeated it." We ended every communion prayer by stating, "I am healed and whole in the Name of Jesus, Amen."

As we obeyed scripture and connected our hearts to Christ in this sacred, spiritual act, our connection as a couple also became stronger. "Shepherd, Be Lifted High" by David Funk became our "communion song." To this day, I can hear even just the intro, and it takes me right back to those precious moments of Jonathan and me seeking healing through communion. With both of us relinquishing our pride and humbly praying together in agreement with God's Word, our communion time unleashed a new power in our marriage. "Where two or more are gathered, there He is in the midst of them" (Matthew 18:19-20). We knew that God was present with us every single time, and we still do it regularly today.

If you haven't already, I encourage you to start incorporating communion into your healing journey immediately. Jesus wants to spend that time daily with you. He told us in Luke 22:19, "Do this in remembrance of Me." Take a step of faith and let this become a sacred time for you, just as was for us. Make room for His healing power to flow in every area of your life!

While waiting those two weeks for my next appointment, we continued to pray, worship, and take communion, while also maintaining our busy schedule with five kids, and trying to maintain our privacy about everything. It was a lot to juggle but our priorities were set. We set aside lots of time to pray and reflect. Thankfully, our small but strong support network of prayer warriors checked up on us often and sent encouragement regularly. Grandma Hunt would come over with her Bible and other study materials, and would pray with me and fought the enemy for my life. She taught me how to pray with authority, how to declare healing through words and how to rebuke pain and cast out fearful thoughts. I will be passing these things along to you more specifically throughout the coming chapters. I'm so thankful Grandma knows the Word of God intimately, and always shows up ready to pray and ready for spiritual warfare. I treasure everything she taught me.

Take a Step of Faith

1. Are you ready to disown your diagnosis? If so, say this out loud:
    "_____(diagnosis) you have no right to my body. I choose to believe the report of the Lord which says I am healed in Jesus' Name."

2. Have you ever taken communion personally in your own home? It doesn't have to be anything formal. There's power in remembering and honoring what Jesus did for us on the cross. Today, find a cracker or a piece of bread and some juice or wine. Say a prayer, forgive anyone who has offended you, and thank God for His covenant with us!

3. Do you have a trusted prayer friend in your life? If not, can you think of someone you know who you could ask? Pray and ask God to make it clear. He does not want you to walk through this alone, and He will bring the right people into your life.

CHAPTER 2

Reflecting on Past Testimonies

I wish I could tell you that my faith was always strong and unwavering as I waited for that upcoming CT appointment, but truthfully, I had to wrestle with my mind daily. The diagnosis consumed my thoughts. Notice that I call it a "diagnosis," not "my cancer." It was an unwanted trespasser in my body. I did not want to identify with it or give my body permission just to accept it. I needed my body to stay in a posture of resistance which starts by keeping my mind in a posture of resistance. If you have been diagnosed with any sickness or disease, make sure you are not claiming it or speaking it over yourself. You do not "have cancer." That may be a diagnosis you received, but it does not belong to you, and it does not belong in your body. Although the diagnosis may be scientifically accurate, don't take it on as your identity. We must first change the mindset of "having" a disease because that directly contradicts healing. There is not one thing Jesus hasn't already defeated on the cross. He paid the price for cancer and all diseases. If you are in the habit of saying, "I have cancer," you must stop immediately. Stop cursing your own body. When speaking of it, say that you've been diagnosed with it, but never again say "my cancer." If you accidentally slip, catch yourself and break that curse out loud. "I rebuke that. I do not have cancer; it is not mine. I am healed, in the Name of Jesus."

Because cancer was my war, I tend to speak specifically to that, but the same principles apply to any sickness or disease. Just as I could not allow myself to identify as a cancer patient, you cannot identify as a recipient of cancer, heart disease, lung disease, kidney disease—it does not matter the diagnosis. Say out loud, "I am not a victim of _____, I am healed in the Name of Jesus!" It may feel strange at first, just like it felt strange for us to take communion. But go ahead and get into the habit of saying it out loud. Tell yourself the truth, and you will believe the truth!

I mentioned the power of sharing testimonies for the sake of others, but there is also something powerful about keeping an account of testimonies for ourselves. It keeps our faith fresh and alive and serves as a constant reminder of how faithful God is. Sometimes other people need to hear our testimonies, and sometimes we need to hear them ourselves. To help calm my racing thoughts, I began reflecting on all the ways God had been faithful to me in the past. Doing so was a powerful reminder that I could turn to God and trust Him again for this healing. In scripture, David did the same thing. He reflected on his past victories before he faced Goliath. In I Samuel 17:36, he recounts, "I killed a lion and a bear, and today God will deliver this Philistine into my hands!"

In times of doubt and difficulty, I had to consider the evidence of God's faithfulness that I had already experienced. It was like taking my faith to court. I had evidence of His goodness, evidence of His plans to prosper me, to give me a hope and a future, not to harm me (Jeremiah 29:11). I knew that He didn't open doors and "part the Red Sea" in my past, so to speak, only to let me die in this wilderness. So when I needed to encourage myself, I would go back to my gratitude journal that I kept from other painful seasons in my life, and I would spend some time reflecting on what I had written. I recounted the struggles and challenges in my past, and the impossible situations I had faced and overcome. I was reminded of how God had already restored my life and blessed me tremendously. He never once failed me and always came through when I truly trusted Him.

I came to a place where I dared to trust God in this circumstance because I already had a history of His intervention in my life. For example, He had already healed my heart from betrayals in the past. He provided for me and restored my finances when I was a single mother and had hardly a penny to my name. He already fulfilled many of His promises from the Bible. He restored what the enemy had stolen from my family. He gave me joy where there was mourning. He showed me that His plans really are to prosper me, not to harm me. He made beauty from the ashes of my life. He made a way for me many times when I faced impossible obstacles. I never want to forget what God has done for me or just how trustworthy He is.

None of us is without testimonies of His goodness. Can you look back and see God at work in your life? Look for the ordinary miracles—the miracle of life and breath. The miracle of the sunrise. The blessing of refreshing rain. If you don't already have a Gratitude Journal or a place to write down testimonies, I encourage you to start today. It doesn't have to be anything fancy. You can leave a simple notebook by your bedside so you can take a few minutes each day to record something you are thankful for. Gratitude is a powerful force, and it is the first block in the foundation for my healing journey.

Over the following pages, I want to share with you some testimonies of what God has done in my life. These are the stories that fueled my faith to believe that God would be faithful again. I pray they inspire your heart as well. Revelation 12:11 says, "We overcome by the blood of the Lamb and the word of our testimony." We can never underestimate the power of giving testimony to the glory of God!

Testimony of My Daughters

Even though I am young, I have been married before. Triplets run in my family, and believe it or not, in my former marriage, my first pregnancy was triplets. Conceived naturally. This was a wonderful, unexpected blessing, but it was a pregnancy that came with risks. I was overjoyed and overwhelmed all at the same time. Once I discovered I was carrying triplets, I prayed for three happy, healthy babies with no complications. I also asked God to help me carry them to 34 weeks, which is the ideal time for triplets. Thankfully, I delivered three beautiful baby girls at exactly 34 weeks gestation to the day—no complications, all happy and healthy with minimal interventions. They all went home after a short two-week stay in the NICU (neonatal intensive care unit), and looking at them now, you'd never guess they were ever preemies or that their birth was considered high risk. Cameron, Courtney and Chelsea are happy, healthy, beautiful gifts from above.

It still fascinates me to this day that God chose to give me triplets. He knew how much joy they would bring to my life. He knew me before I was even formed in my mother's womb, and He already created me to be a mom of triplets! He had already equipped me with everything I needed to raise them, and I have adored every single moment of motherhood. I cannot imagine my life without having all three at one time. It is truly such an amazing blessing that few get to experience.

Testimony of the Healing of My Heart

When the girls were four years old, I gave birth to my fourth daughter Alaina, right in the middle of the tragic ending of my first marriage. I was delighted by her birth but devastated by my divorce. I remember saying aloud, "God Himself cannot heal me from this pain and betrayal I feel." At the time, it was the most painful experience I had ever been through, but God has an amazing way of taking tragedies and turning them into blessings.

Over the years that followed, I began healing and rebuilding who I was and what I believed. I grew in my faith and experienced a deeper love and trust for God. I began to see Him as my Provider and Protector, the One I could truly count on—not just the all-powerful God we worship in church. My relationship with Him became more personal, and I was finally able to trust Him with my future, something I regretted not doing sooner. In my younger years, I would just "tell" God what I was planning and then ask Him to bless it. Looking back, that seems incredibly ridiculous and foolish. Now, I ask Him what His plans are for me so that I can follow what He wants. I know His plans are already blessed! I could have saved myself years of regret and consequences had I just turned to Him and trusted Him first. Now, I have experienced firsthand how God can give beauty for ashes, joy for mourning and a garment of praise instead of a spirit of despair (Isaiah 61:3). I experienced what He meant when He said, "I will restore to you the years the locust hath eaten" (Joel 2:25). This verse tells us that when we have a season of destruction, like locusts eating a beautiful harvest, God promises to restore that harvest back to us.

Testimony of His Love for Me

During the season after my divorce, as a single mom with four daughters, I experienced challenges in dating, but mostly because I did not see value in myself. Although relationships require compromise, I was leading with my hurt and loneliness. I kept compromising on the wrong things and tolerating character issues that were against my values simply because I did not want to be alone. For example, I was in a committed relationship with a man who told me he'd "marry me tomorrow" if it wasn't for my kids. His reservation was because if I ever had issues collecting child support, he didn't want to spend his hard-earned money taking care of my kids. That was incredibly painful to hear. In fact, I didn't want to hear it, so I told myself that he didn't really mean it. I convinced myself that if we stayed together long enough, he would learn to love my daughters as his own. It seemed a better option than moving on because for a while, I believed that no man would want the package of a mom with four kids. But as time went on, things did not change with him and I had to make a hard decision. The final straw was when we went out to eat at a restaurant with the girls for the first time. He and I had been dating a while, but the children always stayed behind with a babysitter. When the bill came, this man offered to pay for my meal, but he told the waitress to put my children's meals on a separate check so I could pay for them myself!

Although I was able to forgive him for his rude and shameful treatment, it was much harder to forgive myself for having such low self-esteem that I tolerated this type of behavior for even a second. The brokenness from my previous relationship left me doubting my self-worth. I had not discovered my value and identity in God at that time. I had not fully accepted that I was worth receiving the best promises that God has to offer. I often felt like a beggar asking God for things I wanted, because I felt so unworthy. I didn't know that I should come to His throne boldly as a daughter of the King of Kings. But after that experience, I was motivated to pray that God would bring me a man with a generous heart, who would love my children like his own and not view them as a financial burden. I started praying this prayer even though I hadn't formally broken off the relationship yet! By this time, I had regained financial independence working as a massage therapist. I did not need anyone else to financially support me or my children, but I wanted to be with a man who would love them like his own and enjoy their presence. I wanted someone who would make them feel loved and valued, and treat them like the daughters of heaven that they truly are.

Shortly after that terrible dinner out, I was at work when a new patient came in for a massage. I was supposed to start our session by asking her intake questions about where her pain was located what she would like me to focus on during the massage, etc., but she started asking *me* all kinds of personal questions, specifically about my dating life! "Are you married? Do you have children? Who are you dating? Does he love your children? Why are you unhappy in this relationship?" Her questions hit the core of what I was feeling and had me in tears. She said "Honey, I feel like God sent me in here today to talk to you." She was in her 80's and full of Godly wisdom. It was clearly a divine appointment. We became very close as she became a regular patient of mine. I enjoyed chatting with her as she always had wisdom to impart to a single mother. She encouraged me not to settle in my dating life; she believed that my children deserved the best that God has to offer. She encouraged me to trust God with my future, that He already had a loving husband in mind for me. She encouraged me to write down a list of qualities I desired in a man and to pray over those things. So, I did.

I still hadn't completely broken off that relationship I mentioned. (I know! I know!) I was getting
there, but I was also so confused, broken, and lonely.
To be honest, I was afraid of losing the relationship
I had with his mother, whom I still adore. I remember driving in my car one day and praying about it.
I knew in my heart he was not the right one for me,
but I had been praying for what I wanted and needed
in a man. Was God going to change his heart to fit my
needs? As I was praying, I heard the Holy Spirit speak
to me for the very first time. It was like a downloaded
conversation in my head—a thought I couldn't possibly have come up with on my own.

He said, "Do you think he can take care of you better
than I can?"

That was all I needed, and I knew in that moment
that I was free from that relationship. I knew God was
going to take care of my every need. I did not need to
compromise in my dating life ever again. This was
such a pivotal moment for me. I would not be living
in the full abundance of God's blessings today if I had
not trusted what the Holy Spirit said to me in that
moment. If I had continued in that relationship, my
present would be drastically different than it is today.
This was my first time hearing and following the Holy

Spirit like that, and I have never regretted trusting Him since! Knowing that I could trust Him with my future then, was my anchor for trusting Him to heal me of cancer.

Testimony of Meeting My Husband

For a few months, I prayed consistently over my "list." There were five non-negotiable characteristics I was praying for in a husband and five things that "would be nice" to have but not deal breakers. For the non-negotiables:

1. A man who loves God first.

2. Who is committed and serving in the local church, not someone I would have to drag against his will. (I wanted to see that God was first in his life.)

3. Who would love my children as his own and not see them as burdens.

4. Who is faithful so that I would never have to worry about being cheated on.

5. Who has a strong work ethic.

As for the five things that I simply desired:

1. For him to be a respectful gentleman, classy and well-spoken.
2. That he would be physically attractive to me.
3. That he would love to travel as much as I do.
4. That he would be taller than me.
5. And, as an added bonus, maybe he would be a musician and play the guitar or drums because I personally found both to be very attractive.

These were quite specific requests, but because I was already in my 30's and because of my life experiences, I knew what I wanted, what I didn't want, and what I found to be attractive. True, godly character was the most important thing to me, but I figured, why not get specific with everything I desire in a husband? Nothing is impossible for Him!

Not long ago, I shared this list with a single friend who looked shocked and horrified that I presented a list to God of what I wanted in a husband.

She said, "You can do that?"

"Yes, of course you can do that! God already knows the desires of our heart. I simply put it in writing and prayed over it. It is absolutely okay to do that," I told her. I made sure she understood that I was not giving God an ultimatum, I was not asking for something outside of His will; I was simply asking Him for my desires; desires that He already knew about.

After that, I had a couple of different dates, but I saw red flags almost immediately with each one. Because I was no longer in the mindset that I would have to settle, or that I wasn't worthy, I dropped them very quickly! I stood firm on the desires God had placed in my heart. I was no longer willing to compromise in a relationship with someone who would not put God first. I prayed about my future husband, fully content to be alone until I found the man God was preparing for me.

About a month later, I decided to join the worship team at church. I had attended for a couple of years and wanted to use my ability to sing and play the piano for God's glory. Around the same time, a handsome, tall, lead guitarist, also single, joined our worship team as well. (What a coincidence!) We noticed each other right away, as the two new, single worship team members. We were both incredibly shy at first and did not say a word to each other. There was the occasional eye contact during practice, followed by insane blushing on my end, like head-to-toe blushing that I could feel and had to turn away! It was so bad my chest would break out in an embarrassing splotchy rash and on top of that, my palms would start sweating! This was not good for the keyboard player, but I managed to make it through rehearsal. For some reason, I would think of him randomly throughout the week, although I knew nothing about him at the time, except he was a handsome guitar player who loved Jesus. I felt this strange draw to him, beyond a physical attraction that I couldn't explain. I had never experienced this before. It did not make any sense.

This continued for about a month or two until I was cast as Mary in the Easter play and Jonathan, Mister tall-handsome-guitar-player, was cast as Joseph. At the first rehearsal, I called him "My Joseph," with no idea that I would eventually include that nickname in our wedding vows. The play rehearsals opened the door for us to begin communicating with words instead of sneaking only blushing glances at each other across the stage during worship practice. (Although that continued as well.) We eventually exchanged phone numbers and began chatting all day, every day. The texts would begin with a "good morning" around 6:00 a.m. and continue throughout the day until one of us fell asleep with the phone in our hand late at night. But he did not ask me out on a date. I couldn't figure out what was going on.

One day when the girls were gone for the weekend, I casually hinted that I was going to the beach by myself after church. He responded with, "I am going to the beach as well, maybe we can meet up?" (Smooth, Jonathan!) I wouldn't quite consider that our first date, but it was an incredible day that I will never forget. It was dreary and misty all afternoon, yet at the same time, it felt romantic, almost like a scene out of a movie. We sat on the sand listening to music and talked for about six hours until sunset. Then he took me out for the worst pizza I've ever had in my entire life; it was burned to a crisp! We still joke about it to this day, but nothing could have made the day any less than perfect to me. We had one more casual "beach date" after that, which was even better than the first. He was so sweet and respectful, such a perfect gentleman, however, I still couldn't figure out if he liked me. To my disappointment, he didn't even hold my hand. I was not used to someone holding back like that, so I wondered if he just wanted to be friends. The next day, I invited him over for dessert and a movie. As we sat on the couch together, finally, he held my hand for the first time and made his feelings known. From that day forward, we were inseparable. As I got to know him over the next year, I discovered that he had every quality I had prayed for in a husband and a dad for my daughters–even my "bonus" requests– he plays guitar AND drums and other instruments as well. It was incredible to see how quickly he and the girls naturally bonded. We felt like a family from the start.

Testimony of God Providing

Every year, our church does a 21-day fast, accompanied with a first fruits offering. In case you are unfamiliar with that term, it is a special offering mentioned in scripture completely separate from the tithe, which is our regular giving towards the work of the ministry. While Jonathan and I were dating, we fasted and gave this offering together and made a list of prayers we were believing God to answer for 2018. One of those was a different career path for Jonathan that would allow him to independently provide for our family (of 6 at the time). I was self-sufficient, but this was a goal of his, and one that he wanted to accomplish before we could get married. We created a budget and a specific number that he needed to make. Three months later, he received an incredible employment opportunity with a starting base annual salary that was almost exactly the number we prayed for, just a tad more. This amount was so specific, we could not deny God's hand in it. He bought my engagement ring immediately thereafter, and we were married that summer.

It still feels like God must have been showing off! He answered everything I prayed for in a man. He even gave him an abundance of musical gifts, plus many qualities that I didn't even know I needed. Most importantly, Jonathan has always placed God ahead of me, and I love him for that. I have never known a more loving, intentional human being in my life. He is a better father to my four daughters than most biological fathers I know. He has taken the time to learn their love languages; he is aware of their different emotional needs and pours love and attention into each one. He spends one-on-one time with each of them, taking them each on individual birthday dates which is absolutely precious. The triplet dynamic is unique. It's easy for them to be seen as a group instead of as individuals. They need and crave individual attention probably more than a singleton since they have had to share everything since birth. Jonathan has helped me teach them all that they are daughters of the King, each with unique gifts and abilities, and they deserve to be treated as such. He has set a high standard so that when they are ready to date, they will not have emotional voids or low self-esteem, leading to low standards or settling. He has set the example of how a husband is to treat his wife, loving her as Christ loves the church and putting only God above her. I could write an entire book about all of his amazing qualities alone, but the point of this story is that God restored everything I thought I lost with far better than I ever imagined was possible! I had no idea that marriage could be so wonderful.

For any single ladies or single moms reading this, know that God is the best matchmaker out there. You do not have to settle! Let me repeat, you do not have to settle! When you pray over your future spouse and put your dating life in God's hands, He will not disappoint. You and your children deserve the best that God has to offer. (This goes for the men, too.)

Testimony of Answered Prayer for Jonathan

Although we already had four kids we were raising, we wanted to have one together. Jonathan's desire was to have a son. The most Christlike love I had ever seen or experienced was his love for me and my daughters, and because of that, I had no doubt that God would honor the desire of his heart and give us a son. Months before I even got pregnant, I began buying baby boy clothing in faith. Then, in September of 2019, I found out that I was expecting. I did not pray for it to be a boy; I just knew in my heart that it was. And in June of 2020, our son, Jacob, was born. God is so faithful to our needs and desires again and again!

As you can see, I have just too much evidence of God's faithfulness in my life to think He would give me cancer or fail to heal me of it. He's just too good, and He always comes through for me when I trust Him. I was thankful that I had documented all these testimonies, and I have so many more. As I reflected on these specific ones, I came to certain absolute, undeniable truths:

1. God did not restore my life to have it ripped apart now. He did not work that miracle of bringing such a loving husband and father to me and the girls, just to let me die. Since Jonathan is not their biological father, if something were to happen to me, he would have no legal rights to them. God undeniably brought him into their lives. He did not do that just to have our family torn apart now.

2. He also didn't open doors and career opportunities for Jonathan to provide for his family, only

to have his new family torn apart by death.

3. He did not work out this incredible act of restoration yet plan for me to have a radical hysterectomy, which would send me into menopause immediately as a newlywed.

All of the evidence told me that cancer was not a diagnosis or a curse from God. My past testimonies prove why cancer was not God's plan for me, and neither was a radical surgery. But this would not be a one-time conversation with myself. I had to remind myself of these truths all day, every single day. Some might say I was in denial, but I say that I was in acceptance—acceptance of God's healing. As an act of faith, I decided to start writing my new testimony before I had any evidence of healing. I opened my iPhone notes and wrote "Healing Testimony." I simply started with two dates, the biopsy date and the diagnosis date, the rest was blank. I waited and believed for the testimony part to come.

Take a Step of Faith

1. Did something in these testimonies resonate with you? If so, which part?

2. Is there an area of your life where you are settling for less than God's best? Are you willing to let it go and see what God will do in your life?

3. What are some of your testimonies you have of God's faithfulness?

4. Do you have a gratitude journal? If so, make sure to review it often. If not, today is a good day to get one started!

CHAPTER 3

Holy Spirit Intervention

Waiting is not something I particularly enjoy. In fact, I seldom wait in line for anything if I can avoid it. I order food ahead on various apps, so it's ready when I arrive. I even order my groceries ahead of time and have them delivered to my home. I love the conveniences of modern technology. But here I was, waiting for the CT scan, waiting for the appointment with the oncologist, waiting for God to heal me. There is no way to "call ahead" or put a rush order in with God. This period of waiting was so hard for me. In fact, I was miserable. Every day of the waiting period was just emotionally draining. I was feeling so overwhelmed by everything. Even when my faith was strong, it was still an uphill battle to keep it that way. I initially had thoughts of canceling everything on my schedule. I wanted to spend every minute with my family. I also just wanted to cry when I needed to, to pray and fight this battle in the privacy of my home, and not feel the pressure to "put on a happy face" in front of the world. But there really wasn't much that we could cut out of our schedule without raising suspicion with the kids. We had no intention of even telling them anything until this was all over.

Volunteering on our worship team at church was the one thing that was absolutely not an option to cut out. Jonathan and I still serve regularly in almost every service. He plays the lead guitar, and I play the keyboard. We are both called to do this, and we were not about to let the enemy steal our worship. The Bible tells us that worship is a weapon. Second Chronicles chapter 20 recounts the time Jehoshaphat headed into battle and appointed men to sing to the Lord, sending them out ahead of the army. Scripture states that God fought the battle for them and defeated their enemy. They won because they put God first through their worship. So, it seemed like a nobrainer to us—we were not cutting out worship. Instead, we were going to glorify God through our battle. In fact, we cranked it up a notch. In addition to our two Sunday services, Wednesday service, and rehearsal once a week, we also had worship music playing 24/7 in our home.

There are many places in scripture where the people of God went to battle, and the worshipers went out first. For example, when Joshua fought the battle of Jericho. (Joshua 6) God commanded the armies to march around the city, with the worshipers out front. On the seventh day, they were to blow the trumpets and give a shout of victory! When they did as God commanded, the walls of Jericho came down.

In Psalm 22:3, it says that God inhabits the praises of His people. Now, scripture distinguishes between the omnipresence of God and the manifest presence of God. Yes, God is everywhere. He is omnipresent. But His manifest presence is different. He manifests in our midst when we worship from the heart, in spirit, and in truth. Very often, we can physically feel His manifest presence in times of worship, and when God shows up, every enemy must flee! This is why worship is so important in the life of the believer.

So, I made a playlist called Healing Inspiration, filled with songs of God's victory. When I was in an upbeat "fighting" mood, I had a song for that. When I was in a state of grieving, I had a song to provide comfort and remind me of God's faithfulness. When I was feeling anxious, I would play a song to give me peace. Worship music is so powerful that when King Jehoshaphat sent the worshipers out ahead of the army, God fought the entire battle for them, and not one of their enemies escaped (II Chronicles 20:24). You can worship your way into a victory! I highly recommend finding worship songs that inspire or comfort you and listening to them as constant reminders of God's faithfulness.

A Divine Prayer Appointment

Almost two weeks after my diagnosis, Jonathan and I were with the kids at the Wednesday night youth service at our church. In the middle of service, I got a text from one of my closest friends and prayer warrior, Nickie. A prayer warrior is a person who goes to war in prayer, and who uses the Word of God as a weapon. "The Word of God is living and powerful, and sharper than any two-edged sword, piercing even to the division of soul and spirit, and of joints and marrow, and is a discerner of the thoughts and intents of the heart" (Hebrews 4:12). A prayer warrior knows this and uses God's Word as a mighty weapon, the strongest weapon available to mankind. Grandma Hunt and Nickie are both powerful prayer warriors, and I'm so thankful to have them in my life.

This particular evening, in her text, Nickie asked if she could pray with me after the service. Jonathan and I had driven separate cars to church since he came straight from work, so he agreed to take the kids home so I could stay behind to talk with Nickie.

The time right after service is usually a busy time of fellowship and talking, so it took a bit to get the kids together and loaded into Jonathan's car. What is so interesting to me about that night, is that by the time she and I finally met up, the church was locked up, and almost everyone was gone. We walked out to the parking lot and got into her car, and she turned on the worship song, "How Great Is Our God." It was already a holy moment, and she anointed me with oil and began to pray fervently, declaring healing over my body, rebuking and casting out cancer in the Name of Jesus. She prayed, speaking in tongues and taking authority against this attack from the enemy. She commanded Satan to loose me, declaring that he had no authority to steal my life or health and to let me go. She commanded cancer to leave and spoke life and healing over me. I felt the Holy Spirit touch me right there, in the car, in the middle of an empty church parking lot. As she prayed, both of us were sobbing uncontrollably as we felt the unmistakable warmth and weightiness of the presence of God hovering over us. I suddenly had a physical feeling that the hand of God was directly on my head. Just as I became aware of the sensation, Nickie said "Mandi, the hand of God is on you right now." I have felt the presence of God many times in my life, but this time, it was different. It was more personal than ever before. It was so amazing and wonderful. I would relive that moment every day if I could.

When she finished praying, I said, "I think I was just healed!" I typed it into my phone notes, and rushed home to describe to Jonathan what had just happened. When I got home, the kids were all in bed and I ran straight to Jonathan, looked him in the eyes, and said, "I was healed tonight." I told him about the entire encounter in Nickie's car, and how amazed I was that God touched me and healed me in the empty church parking lot! Jonathan agreed in faith with me; we both declared that I was healed. I wrote it on the chalkboard calendar in the hallway, and I documented on my iPhone calendar. There was no doubt in my mind that I was miraculously healed of cancer on September 8, 2021.

The very next day happened to be my scheduled CT scan. I woke up with excitement, yet thoughts still kept creeping into my mind, thoughts like, *that wasn't really God. What if He didn't heal you?* I had to cast those out. I had to choose different thoughts. I still felt waves of uneasiness, but I had true joy for the first time since the diagnosis. I believed with all of my heart that I was healed.

My appointment was early in the morning, and I somehow got the results back that same afternoon. My results were all within normal limits and there was no cancer identified! I began rejoicing, God had done it! I had received my miracle, there was no cancer found in my body. I was ready to share my testimony and shout it from the rooftops! God had come through for me again; this was truly a miracle! We were in a state of rejoicing, but I still had a follow-up appointment with the oncologist in a few days. I thought about canceling that appointment since I did not have cancer and now had a clean report to prove it, but I decided I would still go and let them know God healed me.

Up until this time, I had refused to research survival rates of adenocarcinoma cancer. But now, I wanted to know just how incredible this healing was, so I started searching things online. I even broke out my old nursing textbooks and read up everything I could find. It was truly incredible that God had healed me of such an aggressive cancer. The survival rates, depending on staging, are not good. Five-year survival rates for localized adenocarcinoma of the cervix is

92%, regional is 58%, and distant is only 18%. It made me sick to read that, but I was also overwhelmed with gratitude to be healed of something so aggressive.

Even though I had a clean report, I still dreaded the appointment. I thought to myself, *I do not belong in an oncology office.* On the drive over, I kept thinking, *one hour max and this will all be over. The doctor will agree that I don't have cancer and that I don't need to be here. Things will go back to normal, and this will be my testimony.*

Jonathan went with me, and when we finally made it back to my appointment room, the doctor and her nurse practitioner were both very nice and professional. I just stayed as quiet as possible. I was so ready to get out of there! "Your CT results look good. We're going to do a pelvic exam today to see what we find," she said. I reluctantly complied, anything to get the appointment over with so I could bolt out of there. As they began the exam, I heard them talking about "it" and estimating a measurement, and I can't even remember what they said beyond that. One of them said, "It's 1.2 centimeters," and the other agreed. I initially thought maybe they were talking about the biopsy scar, but then I received unfathomable news. They both saw the tumor and estimated it was about

1.2 cm wide. I did not understand what I was hearing. God had touched me; I knew I was healed and they couldn't take that away from me!

I began to tell them, "We prayed for God to heal me, and He did. How did my CT scan come back perfect if there is a visible malignant tumor still inside of me?" I asked if she was sure.

"It is adenocarcinoma; it's a very obvious, unmistakable cancer on your cervix," said the oncologist, concurring with the original biopsy report. Having been in practice for close to 30 years, she was an expert in her field and easily able to identify cancer. She also explained that a CT scan would only pick up the cancer if it had spread, and this tumor was too small to be seen on the scan. She diagnosed me with stage 1B adenocarcinoma of the cervix.

"We don't know how deep it goes. We'll have to get an MRI to make sure it's under 4 cm, or the staging will go up."

I began to cry softly, determined not to ugly cry or allow myself to feel defeated. Then she told me, "This is good news that it was caught early. Right now, surgery is an option. But if it's over 4 cm, then I wouldn't even operate; you would need chemotherapy or radiation. So, in the scheme of things, this is good news.

We just have to wait for the MRI."

Hearing this news was even harder than receiving the first vague diagnosis. I walked in there believing I was healed. Now I had one treatment option—a radical hysterectomy with removal of both ovaries. And that was only if the tumor was under four centimeters. This procedure had the best survival rates. However, it would also send me into menopause immediately at 38 years young! I learned that adenocarcinoma is a cancer of the glandular cells (mucous membranes) and statistics show that once it spreads, the survival rates go down drastically. It is a very deadly cancer if not caught very early. This is why being staged as only a 1B that could most likely be treated with surgery was presented as "good news." However, the doctor could not guarantee that I wouldn't also need chemo or radiation if it had spread even to my lymph nodes. I felt sick to my stomach. I wanted to cry, vomit, perhaps both. She wanted to see me back in two weeks, which would give me enough time to complete the MRI. In two weeks, if the tumor was under 4 cm, I would need to schedule a radical hysterectomy. I left that appointment feeling more confusion and fear than I could handle. I wanted desperately to slip into a coma and wake up when it was all over, but that wasn't an option.

Jonathan again proved to be my rock during this time. I was thankful for such a strong, supportive husband who still turned to God for my healing, despite the disheartening news. On the way home, we discussed what the doctor had said, and we decided that we must pray even even more. As we drove back home on the interstate, we played worship music, cried, and poured our hearts out to God. This was beyond our comprehension. We had turned to Him, trusted Him for healing, and believed He had healed me. Yet, here I was with a more specific diagnosis than before and a treatment plan that was horrifying. In my mind, I rehashed the night Nickie prayed for me, and we both knew without a doubt that we felt the presence of God and that I was healed. How was it even possible that there was still a tumor inside me?

I had to go home and play the waiting game again, this time for an MRI. One particular morning, I just wanted to sit and cry privately, and as most mothers know, the only place in the house you can do that is the bathroom. So, I went into my bathroom, locked the door and let the tears flow. Sitting there on the floor, I looked up and noticed the shower needed cleaning. (As most mothers might agree, you might as well be productive even while you are crying your eyes out.) I started to do a quick spot clean, but then I felt this internal nudging from the Holy Spirit to clean the whole shower carefully and thoroughly, the way I want Him to clean my body of cancer. The thought was quick, and I tried to rationalize it. I told myself that was a crazy thought that didn't make any sense, yet I couldn't seem to dismiss this inner feeling. I decided I'd rather be wrong and end up with a spotless shower than ignore the Holy Spirit. After all, I had been begging Him to speak to my heart and give me a word. In my private prayers, I begged for confirmation that I would not die and asked Him to speak directly to me. I needed to hear from Him.

So, I got to work cleaning the shower thoroughly and carefully. At the same time, I was blasting worship music and wallowing in my pity party for one. I was grieving as if I were given a death sentence, which was only the case if I refused the surgery. I was told I could either have a radical hysterectomy or the cancer would spread, and I would die.

Just then, Nickie randomly sent me a link to a sermon she was just watching online and recommended that I watch it right away. I told her I'd check it out, but truthfully, I didn't want to at that moment. I was just being polite. She texted again, "Let me know when you get to 'the part.' You'll know what I mean when you hear it."

So, I reluctantly turned off my music and started this video called, "If These Walls Could Talk," by Sarah Jakes Roberts, and I went back to scrubbing every single inch of my shower. I felt like God was using this chore to teach me something. It was like a metaphor for the sin in my life. He showed me how sometimes there are large, obvious areas of concern that need cleaning. But, as I scrubbed, even in places that appeared clean from afar, close up I kept finding it was dirty. I knew that I needed to get rid of the large sin in my life, but I also needed to search for the less visible sin as well, such as bitterness or unspoken hatred in my heart.

I continued to scrub and scrub and analyze the sin in my life as I listened to the message on YouTube. Then I heard it—the part of the message Nickie was referring to. There was no doubt that it was the confirmation I had prayed for! I burst into tears when I heard the words, "I don't know who needs to hear this, but you shall live and not die. And you will declare that the Lord was working through it all. You shall live and not die. Not 'you shall survive and not die,' not 'you shall barely make it and not die,' but you will LIVE. I hear God saying that you will have life and have it more abundantly, that you will not die. I don't know who you are, but I feel it so strongly in my heart right now that God says 'this is not the end!'"

"It's me, Sarah!" I shouted as if she could hear me through the recording. That word was specifically for me, I knew it immediately! She went on to say so much more that touched my heart specifically. I highly recommend listening to the entire message. By the end of it, I knew for certain that I would not die. God was speaking to me through my chores that day, and He also sent me a very specific word as I had asked Him. He had confirmed that I would not die of cancer, but I would have life more abundantly. I believed it, but I still wondered, *how is this possible?* A radical hysterectomy was not my idea of "life more abundantly." I knew enough to keep my thoughts in my head. Once you start voicing questions, the enemy can use them against you. I just pondered these things in my heart and finished my cleaning for the day.

That night, Jonathan and I took communion as we had every night since Grandma Hunt instructed us to. We thanked God for sending His only Son to die for our sins. As we broke the bread, we remembered and thanked Jesus for allowing His body to be beaten and bruised for our sins. As we drank the wine, we remembered and thanked Him for His precious blood that was spilled. We spoke and declared healing over my body. Every time, at the end of communion, I spoke out loud, "I am healed and whole in the Name of Jesus." Even if I had to say it through tears and fight back doubt, I continued to claim it.

At the same time, I also felt that I needed to make a drastic change in my diet, so I started researching different ways of healing cancer naturally. The Bible says that faith without works is dead, which tells us that we have to do things in the natural that support what we are believing for, so I knew I needed to take action in some way. I wanted to sow seeds of health into my physical being and have some sense of control over my body again. I heard about a remarkable program by Chris Wark of chrisbeatcancer.com and decided to buy a membership. I can't recommend this program highly enough! I did not have the energy or focus to do extensive research on food and anticancer regimens and, Chris Wark, the founder, already did the work and organized it into an easy-to-follow plan. We ordered a juicer, and I started this radical diet change called Square 1. I didn't want this to be just a diet though, I was feeling convicted to fast on some level. Jonathan was so supportive and decided to do the program with me as a way to fast and consecrate ourselves to God. We both committed to at least a month. I started on September 27th; then we committed the entire month of October.

Three days after I began the juice fast, I went in for my MRI. While sitting in the waiting room, I was filling out my paperwork, and I had to check a box that asked whether or not I had cancer. I sat and stared at the box, struggling with how to answer that question. I was there for an MRI because I had a cancer diagnosis, but I was not willing to claim it. Instead I was claiming what God says about me—that I am healed and whole in Jesus' Name. I debated heavily with myself and then rationalized it all in my head. *Since cancer is what they are to be looking for in the MRI, perhaps I need to answer "yes."* I marked the "yes" box and immediately regretted it. I felt that even though I had broken the curse of cancer out loud, I just contradicted myself, and now I was claiming cancer on paper. So, I quickly marked it out and checked "no" instead.

When the tech took me back for the MRI, she was confused by my paperwork and asked me for clarification. I explained to her with tears in my eyes and a shaky voice, "A biopsy revealed cancer recently, but I'm here today for confirmation that God has healed me." She seemed a little shocked, and I'm sure I must have sounded half crazy to her, but she was sweet and encouraging. Then, I asked her if I could play my worship music during the MRI. Although she told me the machine would be too loud to hear, I chose to play it anyway. I wanted words of victory and worship filling the room and setting an atmosphere of peace around me.

A few days later, they scheduled my review with the oncologist. The night before my appointment, I was scheduled to sing for what we call "Hunger Night" at our church. Hunger Night is a night of worship and prayer where people can come and fill the deepest hunger in their spirits for God. When the service was over, I asked two of my dear friends if they would pray for me. Nickie and Dolly anointed me with oil and began to pray. This time, the Holy Spirit spoke a word through Nickie; a word meant for me; a confirmation of my life and a message that still brings tears to my eyes and quickens my heart.

She said, "The Lord says, 'As I'm cleansing you of cancer, I'm cleansing your heart of past shame and guilt that you've held on to. It will not be delayed.'" Her words pierced my heart, and my eyes flooded with tears. God indeed was using all of this to show me that He was doing a deeper work in me than what

I could see on the surface.

When I think back, those words still prick my heart. My Creator told me that He was healing me, and it would not be delayed. That was a truth that I would hold in my heart as an anchor over the months that followed when everything I believed seemed to be contradicted by the doctors. Nickie also confirmed other assignments in my life, speaking of gifts that God had given me and His future plans for me. It was an incredible, beautiful moment for which I am thankful. God knew the fears I was battling, and that I was trying to keep my faith strong. He knew that I trusted Him more than the doctors, and showed me mercy and compassion. He didn't have to give me that confirmation, but He's just that merciful. I left church that night with a new confidence.

The next day, Jonathan and I went to my appointment with the oncologist. I walked in feeling like a completely different person than who I was when I walked out of that same office exactly two weeks prior. This time I was confident, not confused. After all, the Holy Spirit had just confirmed my healing the night before. The doctor walked in smiling and cheerful and asked if we had seen the results of my MRI. "It came back perfect, there was no cancer detected on the scan," she said. Jonathan and I made eye contact; we knew exactly why it came back perfect. She had a slightly perplexed look on her face and said, "You don't have a pelvic exam scheduled today, but would it be okay if we take a look?" I consented as I had already planned to ask for another exam. I needed confirmation that it was gone once and for all.

As I was laying there being examined, I heard the doctor and nurse practitioner chatting. "It looks different," one of them spoke in a perplexed voice. The other agreed, "Yes, let me take another look." I asked if that was a bad thing, to which they responded, "No, just different." During my first exam, they measured the visible part of this malignant, high-grade, rapidly dividing, rapidly spreading, aggressive tumor at 1.2 cm and they hoped that the entire tumor was less than 4 cm. Instead, it didn't show up on the MRI at all, and they measured it at only .5 cm that day. I was so excited to hear that news. I exclaimed, "It shrunk!"

The conversation that followed was almost comical. Just the night before, the Holy Spirit had said that He was cleansing me of cancer, and it would not be delayed. This was evidence of His word.

The doctor responded, "No, I wouldn't say it shrunk,

it just looks different." I could not believe my ears.

"How big did you measure it today?" I asked.

Now, I'm no math genius, but I do know without a doubt that .5 cm is smaller than 1.2 cm, I thought.

"When I was here two weeks ago, you measured it at 1.2, but today it's only .5 cm. We prayed for God to heal me, and He is doing just that!"

The doctor still would not agree that the tumor had shrunk. I think she did not want to offer me any false hope. She kept insisting that the area around the tumor looked abnormal and the cancer was still there, and visibly measurable. I of course emphasised that it was less than half the size it was 2 weeks ago. As the appointment continued, I had to keep my focus on the evidence that God was showing me. The doctor still recommended a radical hysterectomy, with no option of keeping my ovaries. I simply could not understand this.

I was firm in my resolve as I told her, "God is healing me, and the measurement today is evidence. I don't want the surgery." She was a very sweet and compassionate doctor, but since she could still see the cancer, that was the only procedure she was willing to do. She sent out referrals to two different doctors who might be willing to do a less radical procedure, although the success rates are lower. I had to leave that appointment holding on to the word from God and not the word from the doctor. As I checked out at the front desk and made my next follow up appointment, I asked the receptionist, Nicole, "Did you see the good news on my paperwork? God is healing me, and the tumor has already shrunk in half." I did not care if the doctor agreed or not. It was basic math, and there was documented proof! I felt the need to go ahead and give God the glory. Nicole began raising her hands in praise and squealed out loud. She was so excited that she almost started running in the office! I was so excited to have a staff member at the oncology office actually rejoice and recognize God's healing power!

She said, "I'm going to invite you to a prayer group to share your testimony."

"Yes," I told her, "I'd love to come."

I had already told God that my answer was "Yes" to any way He wanted to use me. But this was another leap of faith. I had accepted an opportunity to share my testimony of being healed, and I wasn't even all the way healed yet! But I knew it was coming.

It was months later that I would share my full testimony at her prayer group, where the Holy Spirit spoke to me through a pastor I had never met before. She said to me, "You will write the book." It was the day God inspired the title of this book that you're holding in your hand now. You just never know the ripple effect that happens when you take the opportunity to give God the glory through your testimony!

From the day of my initial diagnosis until the day I saw this evidence of healing, it was exactly 40 days. Forty is a significant number in the Bible, and the first thing that came to my mind was how the children of Israel wandered in the wilderness for 40 years. This had been my wilderness, so to speak. I had spent weeks and weeks absolutely desperate for God to come to my aid. I was no longer just asking and waiting, but I finally had proof that God was healing me. I had evidence.

Take a Step of Faith

1. Are you in the habit of playing worship music as much as you can throughout the day? If not, set up a playlist that will help keep your heart and mind focused on the goodness of God. Here is a list of some of my favorite songs that ministered to me during this season:

Believe For It, by Cece Winans

Another In the Fire, by Hillsong

Battle Belongs, by Phil Wickham

Highlands, (Song of Ascent) by Hillsong

Your Nature, by Kari Jobe

Came To My Rescue, by Josh Baldwin

Evidence, by Josh Baldwin

The Battle Is Yours, by Red Rocks Worship

Something Has to Break, by Red Rocks Worship

The Story I'll Tell, by Maverick City

The Truth, by The Belonging Co

2.   I want to encourage you take some time today
      to listen to the message: *If These Walls Could Talk*,
      by Sarah Jakes Roberts.

Write down anything that speaks to your heart.

CHAPTER 4

Faith - Believing the Unseen

After reading that last chapter, you might think it was smooth sailing from there. I feel somewhat fool-ish admitting that I still struggled at times to keep my faith. I was still fighting and rebuking cancer out loud. I felt like I was still in a battle—a battle against fear now. I had to remind myself of what the Lord had told me. I could not allow fear to cripple me and steal my faith. The Bible says 365 times, "Do not fear!" It is no coincidence that we have that command for the exact number of days in a year. He has covered every day of every year, commanding us not to fear. In the past, I made my worst decisions when I made them from a place of fear. I refused to consent to that rad-ical surgery simply because of fear, but I also did not want to neglect my health.

Other than this diagnosis, I was extremely healthy. Yet somehow, I was incredibly tired all the time. At times, fear would creep in, telling me that it was the cancer causing the tiredness. But deep down inside, I knew that wasn't it. I refused to believe it. But I was so unexplainably tired, I could not survive the day without a nap, and in the evenings, I was ready to go to bed extremely early. I genuinely believe this exhaustion was because my heart and mind were fighting so hard spiritually that my body had trouble keeping up. In the moments of extreme fatigue, I continued to play worship music even when I wasn't physically worshiping. I made sure to fill the atmosphere around me with praise. I made a soft, peaceful worship playlist that I played while I would sleep. These songs were written straight from the Bible, songs of peace, healing, and victory. God's Word is equally as powerful whether we speak it or sing it. If God's Word does not return void and will accomplish what He pleases, then the same is true of His Word quoted in worship songs. Looking back, I may have experienced the most restful sleep of my life during this season!

I had two referrals to doctors who were willing to perform less radical procedures; however, both were declined because neither took my insurance. I found a third facility that was willing to see me, but again they did not accept my insurance, and the out-of-pocket expense was not financially feasible for us. I called a fourth oncology office that would take my insurance, but their top gynecology oncologist was leaving in a couple months, so they were only taking patients on a case-by-case basis. I sent them my health history and exam results for consideration and waited. When the office contacted me, they told me the oncologist had personally reviewed my case and was unwilling to take me as a patient.

So here I was at a "Red Sea" moment. The Israelites in scripture didn't have any options, I didn't seem to have any either. The only doctor who would see me was willing to do one thing—a radical hysterectomy, which is exactly what I did not want. The tears were overflowing again, I just could not understand. I kept going back to what God said, "It will not be delayed." I began to overanalyze everything. *Is God's idea of healing just making enough go away so that I could have a less radical procedure? No, I don't think so. God is not a half-way healer. He didn't get rid of most of the leper's spots, He healed him all the way. He didn't give the blind man some of his sight back, or sight in one eye, but keep the other one blind. So, why is my only option still getting this radical surgery?* I just could not believe that this was God's plan for me. I went back to those absolute truths I mentioned at the end of Chapter 2. This was a defining point in my healing journey.

One afternoon, Grandma Hunt came back over to visit, and I shared everything with her and just cried. Although I believed strongly that God could and would heal me, I was aware of the reality that I didn't get to decide how or when He would heal me. Was I being stubborn and only willing to accept the type of healing that I wanted? Was I wrong for not wanting the surgery and only wanting a miraculous healing?

In the midst of my questions and internal struggle, Grandma asked me a question, "Amanda, what testimony would give God the greatest glory, having the surgery or having a miraculous healing?"

I said, "Of course, a miraculous healing would give Him the greatest glory. I know that He can use a doctor to heal, but I don't want to rely on a surgery for something God has already said that He is healing!" So, Grandma Hunt reminded me of Matthew 9:29 when Jesus said "According to your faith, let it be done to you."

I decided once more, that regardless of what the doctor said, I was trusting God alone to heal me, not surgery. I was believing God for a miracle. So that is what we prayed for right then and there. In the natural, it looked like my only option was surgery, but with God, nothing is impossible. To the Israelites, it looked like they had only the Red Sea in front of them or death behind them. I felt the same way. In the natural realm, the options were either surgery ahead of me, or illness and death closing in. But I knew that God could "part the sea" and do a miracle before my very eyes. I didn't know how, but I knew that my faith would remain in Him. I could not come this far and give up on Him now.

As I waited and kept fighting the good fight of faith, I continued to declare God's promises over my life. I stood knowing that God is bound by His own Word, not mine. His Word says, "By His stripes you are healed" (Isaiah 53:5). His message straight to me was, "It will not be delayed." I had to hold onto these words all day, every day. I prayed and spoke God's Word back to Him, even through the tears.

One of my prayers was, "God, thank You for being true to Your Word. Thank you that I can trust You even when it looks impossible. You are bound by Your own Word, and You said that it will not be delayed. You said that by Jesus' stripes I am healed. Those are Your words, not mine. I am trusting You to heal me. Thank You that the cancer is already shrinking and thank You that it cannot remain in my body. I bind cancer in the Name of Jesus. It is done!" I also spoke every promise of God that I could think of. I claimed that I was all the way healed before I could see it. I refused to schedule a surgery because God had given me more than enough evidence to trust Him.

In the midst of all of this, I had to be aware that God is not bound by time. He is the One who created time, and is outside of it. That's a bit of a headtrip for us as humans because we are so used to quantifying everything in timeframes, but God doesn't do that. I knew He had given me a word, and I wanted Him to heal me immediately. Although He is faithful to His Word and bound to complete what He says He will do, He has no obligation to do it in the time frame that you or I want. Just because I did not see the healing immediately, it does not mean that He is any less faithful. The same is true for whatever you may be waiting for God to do. He will do what He said He would do, but in His perfect timing which may not be your desired timing. That is why we must keep our faith. Hebrews 11:1 says, "Faith is the substance of things hoped for, the evidence of things not seen." Just because I did not see my healing fully manifested at that point in time did not mean that God wasn't healing me. I had to continue believing Him for what I could not see.

Throughout this battle, I had to reject thoughts of

doubt that were trying to make me fearful. Satan is relentless at trying to get us to waiver in our thoughts. If we waiver in our thoughts, we will waiver in our faith. The Bible says in James 4:7, "Therefore, submit to God. Resist the devil and he will flee from you."

I had to resist him over and over. Negative thoughts would creep into my head, telling me that I wouldn't be healed. *What if it just looked like it shrunk in size, but it really didn't? Was it just because the biopsy had healed over? What if the cancer really was still there but not visible under the scar? After all, it did not originate on the outside where it was found. What if it has grown since my last appointment?* I was tormented with these "what if" thoughts from the enemy. Sometimes I would cry because of the intense fear creeping in, then get angry at myself for allowing doubt and fear into my mind. I was angry that it was a struggle, even after God had spoken so clearly and had given me the evidence that I prayed for. I was furious with myself for doubting Him even for a moment. I was afraid that if I couldn't get these fears under control and stand firm on my faith, He might take my healing away. Of course, that is not what the Bible says, but the struggle in my mind was very real.

I wondered, *what if the cancer comes back even worse?*

I needed to escape from these thoughts so I would always circle back to the fact that God cannot lie. He is true to His Word. If God said He will do it, then He will do it! So, I would intentionally meditate on that, and it became a shield for my mind against the fiery darts of the enemy. The hardest part of this entire journey was the war inside my own mind. I did not ever physically see the cancer; I did not ever feel the cancer. I was told it was there, and that is what created the war. Words I heard produced those thoughts in my mind.

If you are experiencing something similar, you have tools and weapons for the battle you face. Remember that God tells us to resist the enemy because he is relentless. He says that faith as small as a mustard seed will move a mountain (Matthew 17:20). I believe that my faith really was only as small as a mustard seed. But that is all it takes.

About two months had passed and it was getting closer to our December vacation time. At this point, I did not want to go to Hawaii anymore. However, parts of our trip were nonrefundable, not to mention that canceling felt like a reaction coming from a place of doubt or fear. Despite my fickle feelings, Jonathan and I kept the trip as planned. This was an act of faith for us that I would be fully healed by then.

As I began to think about the trip and the excursions and adventures, the two I was most interested in were skydiving and cage diving with sharks. *How amazing would it be to skydive over my favorite beach? And to see a shark up close with the safety of a cage in between us, a thrilling, but a safe adventure.* As a little bit of a thrill seeker, I absolutely love roller coasters, sling shots, fair rides, anything that gives me an adrenaline rush, but with a safety measure in place. As I thought of these things, something became abundantly clear to my heart; *how can I put my trust in a parachute, a metal cage, or a safety strap to protect my life, yet have doubts about God's protection over my life? Do I really have more faith in a parachute against gravity, than I do in my God against cancer?* That was an eye-opening thought for me. I had to keep making this decision about faith. Both options before me were unseen—was I going to believe the fear of cancer, or have faith in God? Would I choose to identify with the lies of the enemy or the promises of God?

I began meditating on these thoughts...*I am a child of God, already bought with a price. My life is not my own, my inheritance comes from Him. Not only do I inherit the kingdom, but I inherit the promises of God. The promises that By His stripes, I am healed, He knew me before He formed me in my mother's womb. His plans are to pros-*

per me, to give me hope and a future. The plans of the enemy are to steal, kill and destroy.

There is no doubt, cancer is very clearly not a gift from God, it is not His plan for me. The devastating effects of a radical surgery are not His plans for me. Cancer is a curse from the enemy, a curse meant to steal my joy, therefore my strength, to kill me, to destroy my family. Cancer did not come from God; He already made a way to get through it. Over 2,000 years ago, He sent His only son to pay the price for our healing. Jesus sacrificed His body and His life for all of us, but He would have come for even just one of us. He wants to heal me and you even more than we want to be healed. I had to evaluate whether I believe what God has written and spoken over my life more than what a doctor has written and spoken over my life.

One thing I learned through this entire process is the importance of establishing your identity in Christ. In the natural, the child's identity is based on the parents. A family name shows where you belong. So, to know who you are, you have to know whose you are. Do you know whose you are? If you have joined the family of God by accepting Jesus Christ as your personal Lord and Savior, you are a child of God, a son/daughter of the King. You have been bought with a price and no longer your own. Matthew 7:11 says, "If you, then, though you are evil, know how to give good gifts to your children, how much more will your Father in heaven give good gifts to those who ask Him." God is our Father, and He loves us more than we could ever imagine. When I think of how much I love my own children, I know I would do anything for them. If they come to me asking for something that is good for them, and it is within my ability to provide it, of course, I will give it to them. I may take care of them differently than they expect. As an adult, my ways are different from theirs, because my perspective is different from their young, immature perspectives. I had to see God the same way. He made the greatest sacrifice that could ever be offered, He gave His only Son to pay the ransom for our lives. Jesus endured the worst death imaginable because He loves us so much. The Holy Spirit has returned to be with us, dwell with us, speak to us and guide us. He has shown me that it is God's will to heal me. What a waste it would be if I could not believe enough to receive it.

I was reminded of the woman with the issue of blood in Luke 8:43-48. She suffered from bleeding for twelve years. She had spent all her money on physicians, but no one was able to heal her. She came up behind Jesus and touched the fringe of His cloak, and immediately her bleeding stopped.

"Who touched Me?" Jesus asked the people around him. But they all denied it. "Master," said Peter, "All the people are crowding and pressing against You." But Jesus declared, "Someone touched Me, for I know that power has gone out from Me." He was saying He felt a different kind of touch—a touch of faith. Then the woman, seeing that she could not escape His notice, came trembling and fell down at His feet. In the presence of all the people, she explained why she had touched Him and how she had immediately been healed. "Daughter," said Jesus, "Your faith has healed you. Go in peace."

When I think about this story, it hits me to the core every single time. Jesus mentioned only one thing that made her whole and that was her faith. It was not a list of works, actions, or a certain number of prayers; it wasn't a ritual or list of rules that she had to perform. It was not a level of holiness or sense of perfection. None of those healed her; it was simply her faith in Jesus.

This is a powerful reminder that as we journey through healing, we must keep our faith set firmly in Christ. The woman with the issue of blood did not journey to Jesus thinking that He might heal her, she did not think he was going to heal other people and not her. She knew that if she could just touch His garment, she would be healed. In the same way, we have to know and believe what God says. His Word does not say, "By His stripes, you *could be* healed." It does not say "By His stripes, you *might be* healed"or "By His stripes, He'll think about healing you."It gives no other option but rather states an absolute truth, "By His stripes you ARE healed." Let that sink in for a moment. This leaves no room for doubt. We must have faith in God for our healing. We must be like that woman, who went in with no doubt that Jesus was going to heal her; despite her issue of blood, she made her way through the crowd just to touch His cloak. That is faith at work making a difference!

When you are journaling your absolute truths, write this down and make it personal, "By His stripes, I am healed!" Now say it out loud as many times as it takes for you to believe it. If it takes repeating it 100 times in a row, then do it! You have nothing to lose and healing to gain.

Romans 4:20-21 gives an account of Abraham, known as the father of our faith. It states, "Yet he did not waver through disbelief in the promise of God, but was strengthened in his faith and gave glory to God being fully persuaded that God was able to do what He had promised." God had already promised Abraham a son and that he would be the father of many nations. Even though his wife was past childbearing age, and it looked impossible, he still believed that God was *able to do* what He had promised, but also that He *would do* what He promised. Having faith in God's ability to accomplish what we are asking is not enough, we must also have faith that He is willing to do it. His promises hold true for our own lives.

In Mark 9:23, Jesus says, "If you can believe, all things are possible to him who believes." Let's make that very specific. He said, "...all things." So that includes being healed of cancer. By the time I was diagnosed, I knew that it was His will to heal me of cancer. He bore the stripes 2000 years ago to pay for my healing. So, if I could just believe, then it would be possible for me to be healed of cancer. The same applies to you and any healing that you are seeking. Jesus already said, "I am willing" when He spoke to the leper in Matthew 8:3. He already died on the cross. He told us that He is willing. He died to prove it. He told us that all things are possible to him who believes. Now, believe Him for your healing! He is worthy of our belief and our trust. Numbers 23:19 says, "God is not a man that He should lie, or a son of man, that He should change His mind. Does He speak and not act? Does He promise and not fulfill?" We know that if God said it, it will surely come to pass. We can put our faith in Him; He is true to His Word. He is not whimsical and doesn't change His mind about His promises. He's always reminding us that we can trust what He says. And He says that by His stripes, you ARE healed!

When a health crisis comes our way, we must decide whose words we will believe. Will it be what the doctor says or what God says? Do we hold a doctor and his knowledge in higher regard than the One who created us? Of course not! Now, I'm not at all saying you shouldn't go to doctors or listen to them. We know God uses doctors and medical professionals all the time. The point is that we must not allow a negative diagnosis to open the door to fear. We musn't allow fear to rule our hearts, but rather place our trust in the One who made us, the One who knew us before He knit us in our mother's womb. It's often easy to recognize God as our creator and ruler over all the universe. We believe He is good and in control, but it gets hard to remember that when we face unimaginable trials. I had to remind myself of the following facts:

1. God is our creator and the maker of the Universe.

He is in control. There is no greater power.

2. Jesus paid the price for our healing and died for our sins. Jesus defeated death, hell, and the grave. Every sickness and disease must bow to the authority of His Name. He can even raise the dead. There is nothing He has not defeated already. Cancer is no challenge for Him. He can heal anything in an instant.

3. I have accepted Him as my Lord and Savior; therefore, I am in covenant with Him. A covenant is a binding promise. I am His child and His promises are for His children.

4. He cannot break His Word. If He said He will do it, then He will do it. God is not bound to our word, but bound to His own Word. When we speak His Word (His promises) back to Him, it will not return void, but it will accomplish what He pleases.

5. I believe in unseen things all the time. I never doubt God will give me enough oxygen in my next breath. I never doubt that gravity exists. I trust wholeheartedly every time I turn on a light switch that the light will come on. I may not understand the mechanics of my car, but I make

plans with full confidence that when I'm ready to leave the house, it will start and transport me anywhere I need to go. Is our creator not more trustworthy than the things of the Earth that are forms of His creation in the first place? When it is dark at night, I believe that the sun will rise tomorrow before I see any proof of it. I don't have to see the daylight in advance in order to believe the sun is going to rise today. Healing may be unseen today, but we must believe it is happening just as surely as we believe the sun will rise tomorrow!

6. God wants to heal us even more than we want to be healed. He wants it so badly that He already sent His Son to die, Jesus was willing to pay that price. This is undeniable proof that it is His will to heal.

7. He has said "By My stripes, you are healed." He is trustworthy and He is capable.

Let all of these facts sink in for a moment. Now ask yourself, am I more willing to receive a curse from a doctor or a promise from God? Is the spoken word of a doctor more powerful than the spoken Word of God? Absolutely not. I know God can heal in many different ways, including with doctors and medicine. Each path of healing is an individual journey between you and God, so follow His guidance for your restoration. But know that doctors have limitations, God does not. You do not have to receive a death sentence or an unfavorable diagnosis as the final word over your health.

Speak the Word of God with confidence! You are in a war, and you have the greatest weapon available to mankind, the undefeated Word of God. Nothing can defeat it, not even cancer at any stage. When we speak it, unseen things are happening in the spiritual realm. Battles are being won, the Word of God is defeating the enemy. Satan is relentless because he is powerless. He wants you to doubt God because he knows what will happen when you speak the Word of God against his attacks. It defeats him every single time! Just keep declaring and praising God until you see healing. It will come. Believe for it!

Lastly, don't ignore your emotions. You have the right to be angry! The enemy has come in to steal, kill & destroy. Don't let him win! Take that anger and fight the enemy with God's Word. Rebuke Satan, he cannot have your life. Sickness cannot dwell in you! Jesus paid the price and calls you healed. How dare the enemy to trespass against God's promise!

Take a Step of Faith

Meditate on these words and let this truth sink into your heart:

I am a child of God, already bought with a price. My life is not my own; my inheritance comes from Him. Not only do I inherit the kingdom, but I inherit the promises of God.

The promises that By His stripes, I am healed, He knew me before He formed me in my mother's womb. His plans are to prosper me, and to give me hope and a future.

Over 2,000 years ago, God sent His only Son to pay the price for our healing. Jesus sacrificed His body and His life for all of us, but He would have come for even just one of us.

God wants to heal me and you even more than we want to be healed. I believe what God has written and spoken over my life more than any diagnosis written and spoken over my life.

CHAPTER 5

Forgiveness

I've never had someone take me under their wing the way Grandma Hunt did. Her spontaneous calls and visits were a Godsend. She invested in my health and life in a way that was hard to fathom. She was truly the hands and feet of Jesus during that season. One morning, she came over and talked to me about the importance of forgiveness. Forgiveness isn't something you choose if the person who hurt you deserves it. It's something you choose because God commands it. Forgiveness isn't about letting the other person off the hook; it's about letting yourself off the hook. When you choose forgiveness, you choose freedom for yourself. Let me explain.

Unforgiveness in our hearts becomes bitterness, and scripture tells us that bitterness rots the bones (Psalm 32:3). Unforgiveness is like a spiritual cancer. The Bible says that we need to forgive others so that God will forgive us and hear our prayers.

Grandma Hunt helped me search my heart and deal with any root of bitterness or unforgiveness that did not belong. That was one area of my life I wanted to avoid. There was a lot of pain and betrayal in my past that I had packed away, but Grandma Hunt knew that I needed to deal with it. I tend to be quite guarded in general, perhaps because of what I have experienced, but if I am crossed by someone close, I have a very hard time letting that go. This is a shortcoming that I'm very aware of—no excuses. I can forgive strangers easily, but it is much harder for me to forgive when a person has been close in my life. It wasn't until this moment that I gained clarity on what forgiveness is all about.

At the time, I had carried hatred for someone from my past who had lied, manipulated, betrayed, and deeply wounded me and my children. I knew I no longer had the luxury of avoiding my feelings and holding on to that hurt. It was truly a matter of life or death. Holding this bitterness not only created a spiritual block for God's healing in my life, but even science shows how bitterness and anger makes the body physically sick. My body was baring my bitterness. It had become a cancer in my heart and a cancer in my body. I had to choose forgiveness and not put it off. It was hard because it felt like by forgiving I was letting that person off the hook or that those wounds didn't matter. It felt like I was losing my power, but nothing could be further from the truth. Jesus made it crystal clear how important forgiveness is. You see, forgiveness has nothing to do with the other person and everything to do with you and Jesus. The Holy Spirit was already dealing with me about getting rid of big and small sins in my life, and yes, not forgiving is a sin because Christ commands it. It is directly disobeying Him if we don't forgive. I was at a point where I knew this had to be dealt with quickly. Someone told me, "Forgiveness is setting the prisoner free, then realizing the prisoner was you." I had been in a prison of pain, bitterness, and anger, and it was impacting my health. I wanted to be free, so I turned to the truth of God's Word.

Romans 12:20 says, "Therefore if your enemy is hungry, feed him; if he is thirsty, give him a drink; for in so doing you will heap coals of fire on his head." Coals of fire? *That doesn't sound so bad,* I sarcastically thought. Then I read what Jesus said in Matthew 5:44, "But I say to you, love your enemies, bless those who curse you, do good to those who hate you, and pray for those who spitefully use you and persecute you." And then Matthew 6: 14-15 pierced my heart: "For if you forgive men their trespasses, your heavenly Father will also forgive you. But if you do not forgive men their trespasses, neither will your Father forgive your trespasses."

Forgiveness is God's gift to us. It is the doorway to our own inner healing and the path by which we receive God's forgiveness. I had to decide to forgive, although I still did not feel it in my heart. Grandma Hunt helped me pray a forgiveness prayer out loud and place the entire circumstance in God's hands. That's what forgiveness is. It doesn't mean that what happened doesn't matter. It means that instead of expecting the person who hurt you to heal your pain, you turn it over to God and trust that He will.

Immediately I felt a release in my spirit, but I knew the work wasn't finished. This was just a starting point, but by placing the matter in God's hands, I was saying, "God you be the judge of this person, not me." This would not be a one-time prayer or decision, but it was something I continually prayed until the anger and bitterness was gone.

Another thing I want to mention is that forgiveness is not the same as restoration. Forgiving someone does not mean you have to allow them back into your life. That's completely different. Forgiveness is releasing the pain and bitterness into God's hands.

Don't go back and pick up more hurt and bitterness! Albert Einstein said it best, "Insanity is doing the same thing over and over and expecting different results." Now, God can be healing your relationship too, so you need to lean on Him and follow His peace about which relationships you should invest time in or not.

Another important part of the forgiveness journey is learning to forgive yourself. Have you ever experienced self-hatred? I have so many regrets for mistakes I made in my past—some of which I am still paying the consequences for today. I was mad at myself, and yes, I had to deal privately with self-hatred. I was reminded of Psalms 103:10-14, "He has not dealt with us according to our sins, nor punished us according to our iniquities. For as the heavens are high above the earth, so great is His mercy toward those who fear Him; As far as the east is from the west, so far has He removed our transgressions from us. As a father pities his children, So the Lord pities those who fear Him. For He knows our frame; He remembers that we are dust." I had to receive God's love and forgiveness for myself and let go of the shame and guilt I felt. This cancer diagnosis was not a punishment for them. I have repented, and now they have been cast as far as the east is from the west. What a weight lifted off me!

I came across something interesting in the Bible. Matthew 9, Mark 2, and Luke 5 all give accounts of Jesus healing a paralytic by saying, "Your sins are forgiven." I was desperately trying to get sin out of my life, but I wondered if forgiveness was directly tied to healing. If I have to forgive in order for God to forgive me, and healing is the forgiveness of my sins, then must I forgive in order to be healed? But then I discovered John 9: 1-3, "Now as Jesus was passing by, He saw a man blind from birth and His disciples asked Him, 'Rabbi, who sinned, this man or his parents, that he was born blind?' Jesus answered, 'Neither this man nor his parents sinned, but this happened so that the works of God would be displayed in him.'" When I read this, I thought back to the woman with the issue of blood who was healed by her faith alone. Jesus made no mention of forgiving her sins and I wondered why. Even though I didn't have all the answers, I concluded that no sin was worth holding onto if there was a possibility that it could interfere with my healing. Since Jesus mentioned the forgiving of sins in relation to healing, I believe it's important enough to deal with.

Take a Step of Faith

Now it's time to get honest with yourself. Is there someone in your life you need to forgive? God wants you healed. He wants you to be whole. Forgiveness is the tool to help you be free.

Make a list of anyone you need to forgive and say out loud: "I forgive _____ for _____."

CHAPTER 6

Praying and Speaking

Prior to this diagnosis, I said the majority of my prayers in my head. I know that God heard them because He answered so many of them. Looking back, I am incredibly thankful that He did not deliver the things I prayed for that were not in His will for my life. However, one of the most important, life-altering pieces of advice that Grandma Hunt gave to Jonathan and me was *no more silent prayers*. I remember when she asked us if we prayed out loud together. Until this time, it was rare for us to pray fervently together. So, in her sweet, authoritative Grandma voice, she gave us a suggestion—well, more like a loving command.

"You have to start now," she said. "No more silent prayers. You have to speak them out loud!"

We hold her in such high regard, and if a suggestion comes from her, we know that it is in love, and for our benefit, so we immediately changed how we prayed. We put our pride aside and poured out our hearts together to our Heavenly Father. I can't explain why that was so hard for me, but I had to let go of my pride and pray more in front of my husband. I have never considered myself very good at praying. I have friends, like Nickie, who just bring down the power of the Holy Spirit as soon as she opens her mouth. For some reason, I didn't think that was me. I didn't feel like my prayers sounded eloquent and powerful enough, so I was always reluctant to pray in front of people, including my own husband. I believe this was an area of pride that God wanted me to fix. To some, that may seem strange to call it pride, but I allowed fear of how I thought I sounded to other people, to hinder me from communicating with God and bringing armies of angels to fight for me. In essence, I was making my prayers about how people saw me, instead of how they saw God. That's pride for sure! However, I've now learned the importance of praying out loud together, and I want you to as well. There is power in agreement! Matthew 18:20 says, "For where two or three gather in My Name, there am I with them."

Now, the Bible tells us that we are made in God's image. He created things by speaking them into existence, so we must follow His example and open our mouths and speak. I began to pray like Romans 4:17 and "call those things which do not exist as though they did." Instead of asking for healing, I began thanking God that I was already healed; that all the cancer had left my body. I would not claim even one microscopic cancerous cell. I had to keep my thoughts and my words aligned with what God says. The doctor might have seen cancer last week, but God's Word says I am healed. The doctor might say I need surgery, but God says my healing will not be delayed. The biopsy report might say that there is cancer, but I believe the report of the Lord, and He says that I am healed. I would say, "Thank You Lord that every single cancer cell has left my body. I am healed and whole in the Name of Jesus, and I will stay that way!" I said this many times before I saw my healing manifested, and I challenge you to do the same. You may not have evidence yet that you are healed, but go ahead and begin thanking God before you see it. There is no time in the spiritual realm, and that's why we can thank Him for future events, today. Thank Him and believe Him in advance because it is coming if you believe for it!

Keep in mind that your words have the power of life and death in them. Proverbs 18:21 says, "Death and life are in the power of the tongue: and they that love it shall eat the fruit thereof." What fruit do you want to partake of in your future—the fruit of life or the fruit of death? Are you speaking life and healing over yourself? Or are you speaking sickness and death over your life? If you are claiming cancer (or any other sickness) or calling it yours, then you are receiving that curse and speaking death. If what you are saying disagrees with God's promises, don't say it anymore! You do not have to receive or claim a curse. Yes, anything contrary to what God says is a curse, and you can rebuke it in the Name of Jesus. Just say out loud like I did, "In the Name of Jesus, cancer has to flee. By Your stripes, Jesus, I am healed. The same power that raised Jesus from the dead lives in me. I bind cancer, and it has to leave in the Name of Jesus. I am healed, and whole in the Name of Jesus, and my body will remain whole." You can replace the word "cancer" with anything you are battling.

During my prayer time, I also recalled the lesson of the withered fig tree. In Matthew 21:19, Jesus walked by a tree that was not bearing fruit. He cursed that fig tree, and it immediately withered up and died. In verses 21-22, Jesus says, "Assuredly, I say to you, if you have faith and do not doubt, you will not only do what was done to the fig tree, but also if you say to this mountain, 'Be removed and be cast into the sea,' it will be done. And whatever things you ask in prayer, believing, you will receive." So we cursed cancer and commanded it to wither up, just like the fig tree. We did not hope or wish or think maybe God would do it. We knew He would honor His Word and do what He said He would do. We believed that I was healed before the healing had fully manifested.

Now, the devil is a liar, and he works through deception. He has no authority in the life of a believer unless you give it to Him. As children of the Most High God, we have His authority. We have access to all the power that is in the Name of Jesus! Scripture tells us that every knee will bow, even sickness and disease have to bow to the authority of Jesus Christ. John 14: 12-14 confirms our authority in Jesus Christ. He says, "Truly, truly, I tell you, whoever believes in Me will also do the works that I am doing. He will do even greater things than these because I am going to the Father. And I will do whatever you ask in My Name, so that the Father may be glorified in the Son. If you ask Me for anything in My Name, I will do it." There is a lot in this verse, but it's telling us that if we believe, then we have the authority to cast out sickness and disease just like Jesus did when He was on the earth.

Today, Jesus is at the Father's throne, petitioning for us. If you ask something that is His will in His Name, He will do it! Pray out loud and declare that in the Name of Jesus Christ, you are healed.

Remind yourself of the miracles that Jesus performed. Possibly my favorite one that really spoke to me was in Matthew 8:2-3, "Behold, a leper came and worshiped Him, saying, "Lord, if You are willing, You can make me clean." Then Jesus put out His hand and touched him, saying, "I am willing; be cleansed." Immediately his leprosy was cleansed." Even better is that Jesus went on to be crucified and proved his willingness. He died so that we might live. By His stripes we are healed. He has told us and proven to us that He is willing to heal us. We just have to believe Him and be willing to receive it. Jonathan and I prayed constantly and reminded the Lord of the time He said, "I am willing" and thanked Him for His willingness.

Now, just because we were standing and believing God doesn't mean we disregarded the doctors, and I am not telling you to either. Always follow where God is leading you. We used the knowledge from the doctors as a tool for how to pray. I am thankful for their knowledge and expertise, I absolutely believe knowledge comes from the Lord and He uses doctors, but they do not get the final word! The cross has the final word! And we chose to believe the report of the Lord.

I have to admit, the "what-if" thoughts were still relentless. I remember folding laundry one day and I started having all these terrible thoughts about who my husband would remarry if I died, who would raise my kids, and who would help my daughters get ready on their wedding day. These thoughts tormented me until I did what the Word of God tells us to do. In II Corinthians 10:5 it says to "Cast down arguments and every high thing that exalts itself against the knowledge of God, bringing every thought into captivity to the obedience of Christ." Why do we need to take every thought into captivity? Because thoughts feed our beliefs. The wrong thoughts become the false beliefs. The right thoughts become the right beliefs. I couldn't let those negative thoughts dwell in my mind and become my beliefs.

So instead, I stopped and spoke out loud, "I rebuke that thought, in the Name of Jesus." I took the thoughts captive and replaced them with something that aligned with God's Word, seeing myself healed in my own mind. I imagined myself helping my daughters get ready on their wedding day. I imagined myself spoiling my future grandchildren, and took time to daydream about a long, fulfilling marriage with my husband.

If you are having this same battle in your mind, don't allow yourself to dwell on those thoughts.

Take them captive, speak out and rebuke them. When you resist the devil, he will flee (James 4:7). You have that authority!

God's Word has a purpose in the earth. His words have gone forth, and so our words need to go forth. We need to speak what He speaks. Isaiah 55:11 tells us, "So My Word that proceeds from My mouth will not return to Me empty, but it will accomplish what I please, and it will prosper where I send it." The promises of healing that I declared were not my own. If God recorded a promise in scripture for our use, then it is ours to call back to Him. His Word will not return void.

As I spoke out loud and prayed for my healing, I recalled God's Word right back to Him. I didn't have written prayers that I recited, but in conversation, I told God that I trusted His Word because I knew He could not lie or change His mind, and for that I was thankful. Not that He forgets, but He loves to hear us declare His Word. Like a child going back to their parent to remind them of a promise, I reminded Him that He said His Word never return void and will accomplish what He pleases; therefore I'm healed. I know He won't take back that healing.

No matter what you may be facing today, find specific promises that pertain to your situation and speak them back to God out loud. He says that His own Word will not return void. He told us these things for our own benefit, so declare His promises out loud and watch Him accomplish what He pleases.

Take a Step of Faith

Search the Bible for a promise that speaks specifically to your situation and speak it over your life. Document when you begin speaking it and when it comes to pass.

Begin praying and declaring in the Name of Jesus (if you are not already).

Take a few minutes right now and envision your life on the other side of your healing. How would that change things? What will you be doing? Where will you go? How will your life be different?

CHAPTER 7

Healed

There was one particular miracle in the Bible that I often found entering my mind. The Israelites were trapped at the Red Sea with nowhere to go and an Egyptian army was closing in to kill them. I felt like I was living in my own "Red Sea" moment. I had a doctor who would only do a radical procedure, and others wouldn't even see me. I felt trapped. I needed God to "part the waters," so to speak, to make a way for me, contrary to the path laid out by the doctor.

Sometime in October, I was out running errands one afternoon when I received a phone call from the office of the doctor who previously refused to see me. I was a little annoyed and perhaps short with the receptionist as I reminded her, "The doctor already reviewed my medical history including the biopsy report, MRI and CT I sent over and said she would not take on my case." *How unprofessional and disrespectful for the office to bother me again after they already refused me,* I

WALKING IN THE MIRACULOUS

thought. Before I said another word, the receptionist responded, "She reviewed it again and changed her mind. She does want to see you."

I knew that this change of heart could only have one explanation—God. So, I set up an appointment to see her. I showed up to the appointment and prepared for an exam, with Jonathan by my side for support. This new oncologist had been in practice for 37 years and was quite renowned at a prestigious university in our area. She took her time examining me; she saw the scar from the previous biopsy. She even allowed a resident to do an exam as well. Jonathan and I made eye contact as both doctors diligently examined and searched and finally spoke the words, we had prayed so hard to hear.

"I don't see it."

This obvious, aggressive, rapidly-growing, rapidly-spreading cancerous tumor that had tried to claim me was nowhere to be found!

I had no reservations telling her, "This is exactly what we prayed for! We prayed for God to heal me so I wouldn't need surgery and He did!"

She seemed a little confused and said she wanted to rule out a misdiagnosis. She took two biopsies that day, and ordered in the slides from the original biopsy for review, plus ordered a PET/CT.

I appreciate her attention to detail and diligence in taking my health seriously. Over the next few weeks, she took a total of six biopsies over multiple appointments, desperately searching for the cancer. I was sent for a PET/CT, which came back healthy with no evidence of cancer either. She reviewed the original biopsy slides from August and reviewed the CT and MRI as well. This doctor was extremely thorough and exactly the type of doctor I would want to handle my case. She would not accept a report from another facility. Still, she examined them all herself and had her radiology experts assess them too. Upon reviewing the original slides, she ruled out the theory of a misdiagnosis. She concurred that the original biopsy taken was in fact diagnosed correctly as poorly differentiated adenocarcinoma of the cervix. She submitted my case to the University of Florida Tumor Board for further review and scheduled an appointment for us to discuss the results. When I arrived at that appointment, Jonathan by my side, I had a new peace that is difficult to put into words. I no longer had a sinking feeling as I pulled into the parking garage. I was no longer intimidated or fearful of the word "cancer." I was not unnerved to walk into the oncology office. I was not suppressing tears or feeling anxious waves of nausea. We no longer had difficulty trusting God's Word over a doctor's report. I believed in the unseen more than what I could see. I walked in with complete confidence to hear what the doctor had to say. Let me preface by saying, we had prayed many times for God to show the doctors what He can do, to show them that He is the healer. I believe that He did exactly that.

"The tumor board has never seen anything like this. I can't explain it, I just don't know where it went," my doctor stated.

"I can explain it. God healed me!" I responded.

From there, it seemed like the conversation went around in circles. There had been no cancer in any of my six biopsies, but there were still abnormal cells that could turn into cancer. I once again heard the words "You still need a radical hysterectomy." I could not believe what I was hearing. I argued, "How can you say that when I had an obvious tumor before that you can't even find now? Obviously, God has healed me." Again she stated, "We don't know where it went. Adenocarcinoma is very aggressive and deadly, there could still be something in there, but we won't know until we take out your uterus and send it for pathology."

As she explained the scientific evidence supporting her recommendation, I understood why God had placed that peace and confidence inside me on that very important day. I politely replied, "I appreciate your wisdom and expertise and I understand how aggressive and deadly adenocarcinoma is. But this cancer has done the exact opposite of what science and research say it will do. We prayed, fasted, took communion, and spoke the promises of God, I was anointed with oil and prayed over at our church. I felt the Holy Spirit touch me and He said, "As I'm cleansing you of cancer, I'm cleansing your heart of past shame and guilt. It will not be delayed." And it hasn't. We have watched the tumor shrink and disappear until you can't even find it. I can't ignore what the Holy Spirit told me, or the evidence that He's given me. God has healed me and I'm not having the surgery."

My heart was pounding as I declined the surgery and gave God the glory, yet I felt peaceful. Her words about me needing the surgery and "if there's something still in there" had no weight. They did not ignite fear. She was very respectful about my decision, but chose her words carefully. She referenced my belief that I was healed, but never directly acknowledged that God had healed me.

I have no doubt, I would not be healed today if it

weren't for His healing power and faithfulness to His Word. I have not regretted my decision once. I trust God's Word, not fear. I am healed and whole! God is my radical Healer.

If He Did It for Me, He Will Do It for You

As you can see, I am just an average person who struggles to keep her faith as much as anyone else. It is impossible to earn healing or to ever be deserving of it. But God says you are worth it because He loves you so much. He already paid the price for you to receive it. He sent His only Son to die and pay the penalty of your sin because you are worth it. Jesus bore the stripes because you are worth healing. He gave His life because you are worth dying for. Let your faith allow you to be healed, just like the woman with the issue of blood was healed by hers. Resist the lies from the enemy and choose to believe God. Fight fear by speaking the promises of God.

I want to stress the importance of keeping your faith in God no matter what circumstances look like, even if God does not heal you in the time frame that you want. Keep believing Him and declaring His promises no matter how long it takes. I prayed for an immediate miracle, the way Jesus healed the leper (Matthew 8:3). When I prayed initially, I told God exactly what I needed. I even said out loud to Him, "I'll take a miracle like that. I know You can heal me the way You healed the leper." I had no doubt that He could do it, and I thought that kind of miracle would be best for me. I really believed for that too. I would pray and think about cancer leaving my body immediately. God didn't answer the way I wanted Him to, but He answered in a better way that gives Him even more glory! He was still faithful, and I was able to share what He was doing with so many of the medical staff along the way. If He had answered that request for an immediate miracle, I would have missed many things I learned along this journey and the things that I'm sharing in this book to help you. I would not have changed the way I pray, and I would have missed the experience of seeing what I speak come to life. I would have missed out on seeing His Word fulfilled despite what the doctors said. I would have missed so many opportunities to glorify Him and share this testimony of healing. I believe God will heal in the way that gives Him the greatest glory because He wants to show His goodness to as many people as possible. He wants everyone to come to know Him. I believe that His glory was revealed to so many more people through the way that He chose to heal me rather than the way I was choosing for Him to heal me. Now the entire tumor board at the University of Florida has seen what God can do! Perhaps He used my situation to show some of the doctors who the real healer is.

In retrospect, this four-month journey was not very long, although it seemed like an eternity when I was living through it. I learned so much in such a short amount of time. This curse that came against me actually brought me closer to God and fulfilled His Word yet again. "We know that all things work together for good to those who love God, to those who are called according to His purpose" (Romans 8:28). My faith was tested and strengthened beyond what I thought was possible. I learned to unleash a power God placed inside me—the power of words—to speak life or death, to speak things that are not as though they are, to speak God's promises of healing and see His Word come to pass. Scientific evidence shows that adenocarcinoma is very aggressive. Still everything has to bow at the Name of Jesus, even every variety and every stage of cancer. Ask in Jesus' Name and it will be given to you. I asked for healing in His Name; I spoke God's Word that did not return void. I cursed cancer like Jesus cursed the fig tree and commanded it to wither up. I believed the words that Jesus had spoken over my life! He is worthy of being believed; He already died for us and paid the ransom for our sins. Remember that He loves us and wants to heal us even more than we want to be healed.

If you had asked me the day of my diagnosis if I could ever be thankful for this journey, there is not a chance I would have said yes, I would have done anything to avoid it. However, because of what I have experienced, now I am overjoyed that I have faced the unimaginable, and have a testimony of God's faithfulness. He can be trusted. He is the same yesterday, today, and forever. He is the miracle worker of the Bible, and He is still performing miracles today. He said "I am willing" over 2,000 years ago and He is still willing today. I am so excited to see my children's love and trust for our Creator. They are growing up in scary times, but God has reassured them that He is our protector and our healer. We shared the exciting miracle once the entire journey was over, and they trust Him now more than they did before. To them, He is faithful for healing their mother. My husband's faith has grown too, for God has not only spared his wife's life, but He healed without requiring a surgery that would impact our marriage. Once again, what the enemy meant for evil, God has turned it for good. Every day is a gift, and I'm so thankful to be walking in the miraculous.

Prayer

This is to help you if praying is new to you or you don't know what to pray. Do not rely on reading this word for word, but take these ideas and make it a personal conversation between you and God. It will eventually become more natural to you.

Heavenly Father, I thank You for giving me life on earth and that I get to spend eternity with You. Thank You for sending Your only son to die for my sins and pay the price for my healing. Your Word says that by Your stripes, I am healed. So right now, I claim healing over my body. Your Word says that whatever we bind on earth shall be bound in heaven, and whatever we loose on earth shall be loosed in Heaven. So, I bind cancer in the Name of Jesus, and I release healing. Just as Jesus cursed the fig tree and caused it to wither up and die, I curse cancer and command it to wither up and die. It has no place in my body. My body is a temple of the Holy Spirit, and where Your Spirit exists, cancer cannot stay. It has to flee. Thank You that I am already healed in the Name of Jesus. Thank You for being a man of Your Word, that You don't change Your mind or go back on Your Word. So, I call Your Word back to You, You said it will not return void but it will ac-complish what You please. Jesus, You told the leper, "I am willing" and healed him immediately. Not only did You say that You were willing, but You gave Your life to prove it. So, I receive your healing today. I am healed and whole in Your Name, Jesus. Cancer is not mine, You already paid the price for it, so I give it back to You. I believe what You have spoken over my life, not what the enemy says. You said that Your plans are to prosper me, to give me hope and a future. I receive Your blessings and I rebuke the lies and schemes of the enemy. Silence my ears to his lies and open them to the promises from You. I believe You and I trust You; all my hope is in You. Thank You for dying on the cross and proving just how much You love me. It is finished, it is done. By Your stripes, I am healed. In Your Name Jesus. Amen!

Assignments

1. Begin a gratitude journal. Remember the things that God has already done for you and thank Him. Examine the evidence in your life and find your absolute truths.

2. Establish your identity, and know whose you are. Know that you are a child of God, and His promises belong to you. You are in covenant with Him.

3. Rebuke sickness and disease out loud, and break any curses that have been spoken or written over your life. Stop saying "I have cancer" or "my cancer."

4. Declare God's promises over your life and believe them.

5. Pray out loud. Call God's Word back to Him. Thank Him in advance.

6. Take communion in remembrance of the price already paid for your healing.

7. Take your thoughts captive.

8. Forgive.

9. Praise and worship .

10. Share your testimony.

About the Author

Amanda Hunt is a native Floridian and stay-at-home mother of five (including triplets), married to the man of her dreams. She has her degree in nursing and a background as a massage therapist, but now spends most of her days managing her very full and active household. Together, Amanda and her husband, Jonathan, serve on their worship team at church and in various other ministries with their family.

The Hunt Family

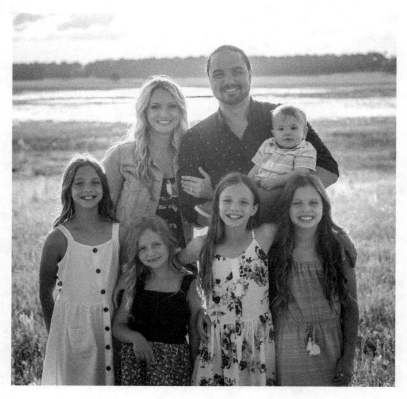

Photo credit: Angel Shaw Photography